An Introduction to Psychiatric Research

When you can measure what you are speaking about, and express it in numbers, you know something about it.

Lord Kelvin, 1824–1907

An Introduction to Psychiatric Research

Richard E. Gordon, M.D., Ph.D.

Department of Psychiatry, College of Medicine
University of Florida

Carolyn J. Hursch, Ph.D.

Psychiatry Department, School of Medicine
University of Colorado

Katherine K. Gordon, R.N., M.A.

Past President, American Psychiatric Association Auxiliary

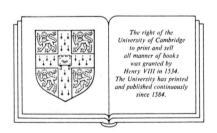

The right of the
University of Cambridge
to print and sell
all manner of books
was granted by
Henry VIII in 1534.
The University has printed
and published continuously
since 1584.

Cambridge University Press

Cambridge
New York   New Rochelle   Melbourne   Sydney

Published by the Press Syndicate of the University of Cambridge
The Pitt Building, Trumpington Street, Cambridge CB2 1RP
32 East 57th Street, New York, NY 10022, USA
10 Stamford Road, Oakleigh, Melbourne 3166, Australia

First published 1988

Printed in Canada

Library of Congress Cataloging-in-Publication Data
Gordon, Richard E.
     An introduction to psychiatric research.
     Includes index.
     1. Psychiatry – Research – Methodology.   I. Hursch,
Carolyn J.   II. Gordon, Katherine K.   III.   Title.
RC337.G67   1988   616.89'007'2   88–2574
ISBN 0 521 35094 8

British Library Cataloguing in Publication applied for

Contents

Contents

Contents   xi

Figures and tables

Figures

Tables

Foreword

A century and a half ago Auguste Comte traced the evolution of human thought through three successive phases, here paraphrased as mystic, quasi-scientific, and comprehensively dynamic. It is significant that psychiatry, a quintessentially humanistic discipline, is only beginning to move past the first two phases. The language of psychiatrists still echoes with reminders of our mystical phase: "Hysteria" evokes Socrates' notions of his shrewish wife Xantippe's misplaced uterus; epileptics (from the Greek *epi-lepsis* – "stricken from above") seem troubled by Jovian "spells" and "seizures"; and "neuroses" are attributed either to malfunctioning neurones (see W. Cullen, who proposed the term in 1716) or to *yang–yin* confrontations between mystic Eros and tenebrous Thanatos (see S. Freud). And it echoes with many more reminders of our quasi-scientific phase: We have adhered to concepts of supposedly discrete "mental disorders," arranged in taxonomies that remained etiologically sterile, semiologically vague, and often prognostically and therapeutically misleading. Despite our currently professed "biopsychosocial" appraisals of individual or group behaviors, we often take as a tenet the centrality of genetic, neuropathological, ecological, or specific experiential influences. We seemed incapable of truly holistic analyses of the polyvectorial etiologies, the protean phenomenologies, and the infinite diversities and permutations of individualized syndromes, each of which requires a skillful combination of biological, psychological, and social interventions. With the possible exception of theology, no discipline spanning study and practice is in greater need of epistemological and therapeutic clarification than psychiatry.

Given this need, *An Introduction to Psychiatric Research* should be enthusiastically welcomed. A glance at its table of contents will indicate its inclusive topical breadth and logical organization. In a clear, precise, reader-oriented style the authors discuss the formulation of heuristic hypotheses, the choice of investigative modalities, the elicitation and organization of relevant data, the statistical tests of their significance, the ethical considerations involved, the derivation of valid inferences, and the lucid reporting of findings in relation to current knowledge and future projections.

The book will be an invaluable guide for mental health professionals already engaged in the disciplined inquiry necessary to move psychiatry into Comte's third stage. It will be particularly instructive for students whose research training will immeasurably improve their contributions to the development of scientific psychiatry, and indeed their services to their patients. The reader is invited to join my literary as well as intellectual appreciation of this major addition to the investigative literature.

> Jules H. Masserman, M.D.
> *Professor Emeritus of Psychiatry*
> *and Neurology*
> *Northwestern University, Chicago*

December 1987

Acknowledgments

We wish to thank the following persons for their assistance. The late Richard Youtz, Ph.D., former Chairman of Psychology at Barnard College, Columbia University, developed the research classification system used here. Richard Gordon, M.B.M., Katherine Reed, J.D., Virginia Ford, B.M.E., and Laurie Gordon-Hardy, J.D., helped gather and analyze data for many of the studies described. Eli Kapostins, Ph.D., of Wagner College, provided excellent critical advice. Khaja Ahsanuddin, M.D., former Chief of Child and Adolescent Psychiatry at the University of Florida, invited us to teach to psychiatric residents the course in research methods that led to this book. Mrs. Gloria Maurer encouraged us to write the book. Roger Burket, M.D., former Chief Resident in Psychiatry at the University of Florida, critically reviewed early drafts of the manuscript. Finally, two clinical psychiatrists, Harvey R. St. Clair, M.D., Area V Deputy Representative of the American Psychiatric Association, and Dan Sprehe, M.D., former President of the Florida Psychiatric Society and current APA Assembly Representative from Florida, provided helpful reviews of later drafts.

We are grateful to the Literary Executor of the late Sir Ronald A. Fisher, F.R.S., to Dr. Frank Yates, F.R.S., and the Longman Group Ltd., London, for permission to reprint Tables III and VII from their book *Statistical Tables for Biological, Agricultural and Medical Research* (6th edition, 1974).

1. Introduction

The purpose of this book

Psychiatry has probably been the least scientific medical specialty. One reason is that its traditional concepts have been hard to measure and its practice has not until recently been quantified and made objective. However, things are changing rapidly. Quantification in clinical psychiatry has grown greatly in the past decade. Researchers have provided clinicians with new concepts and theories and with new tools for diagnosis and evaluation of treatment outcome. As a result, you should not be surprised that organizations that purchase medical services – the government, insurers, employers – are relentlessly forcing psychiatric practitioners to assess and justify their work. Accrediting agencies expect hospitals to evaluate clinical outcomes in patient care as part of their quality assurance programs. The Joint Commission on Accreditation of Hospitals requires practitioners to present evidence showing that treatments are appropriate, efficient, and cost-effective. Younger psychiatrists, especially those who are residents or are beginning practice, will bear the brunt of these demands.

This book will help you to conduct evaluative and other clinical research studies yourself. It also will help you to analyze the scientific literature. It will explain how to tell what credence you can place in a study. Does it follow each research step properly? How do you judge its stage according to the type of question it asks and the tools it uses? What is the reason for choosing a specific statistic? The book will demonstrate how to decide when you need extra help from an expert in your own studies. You need no prior knowledge of statistics or research design to learn from it. It explains the statistical methods used in 97% of psychiatric research (Hokanson, Bryant, Gardner, Luttman, Guernsey & Bienkowski, 1986) and shows how to present and interpret data in correlational or experimental studies.

The book deals primarily with clinical, epidemiological, and nosological studies. It emphasizes the kind of work you can perform in your office with your own patients. It provides you with the statistical tests and experimental designs needed to assess your patients, monitor their progress, evaluate outcomes of therapy, and follow up on patients' subsequent course. You also will learn how to study new scientific tests or equipment that may become available to you and to investigate new phenomena that you may observe – new syndromes or psychiatric responses to unusual events.

Many of our previous publications reported findings from the study of our office patients or patient charts at cooperating hospitals, offices, and clinics. In teaching research methods and writing the chapters that follow, we pursue a similar course: This book uses examples drawn largely but not exclusively from our own studies to illustrate the steps involved in developing research ideas, reviewing and understanding the literature, designing a project, collecting and analyzing data statistically, and getting writings published. It focuses on several themes – stress, socioeconomic position, impairment and disease, social support, coping skills, and functioning.

Some benefits from doing scientific research

To improve patient care. Other medical specialties routinely use X rays, biopsies, biochemical laboratory tests, and the like to demonstrate objectively the necessity for treatment, the kind of care needed, and the effectiveness of therapy. Psychiatry has not routinely used objective instruments to assess patients and trace their progress in treatment, possibly because most psychiatric tests require the use of statistics to determine how much an individual patient or group of patients has been helped by treatment. Yet "objectivity is the single characteristic that sets science apart from all that is not science" (McBurney, 1983). It means simply that other persons would have found the same thing if they had made the same observation. This book describes a number of objective psychiatric tests and provides you with the research methodologies and statistical tools required to analyze and present your findings. The ready availability of the hand calculator and the inexpensive personal computer eases your task of systematically collecting and analyzing data.

The patients you treat often suggest ideas that could lead to improved treatment. For example, you may have the impression that you are treat-

ing significantly more depressed elderly patients and single-parent divor-
cees since you moved from New Jersey to South Florida. If so, are there
implications for your treatment planning? If you keep your patient records in the manner discussed in later chapters of this book and perform
some of the simple statistical tests described, you will quickly answer
these questions. In research conducted with your own patients you can
maintain good control over resources and keep costs down. We performed most of the research discussed here without grant funds and at
little monetary cost. You can conduct similar inexpensive studies in your
own practice.

You can also begin to use new and possibly more effective treatments
with new drugs or new psychosocial approaches reported in studies conducted by others if you know how to appraise the scientific merits of their
work.

Hospital quality assurance committees seek ways of improving patient
care and keeping costs down. They assess patient needs, evaluate programs, monitor patient care, and review the use of resources to accomplish these and other purposes. Their studies employ the research methodologies and statistics described later. You may be called upon to sit on
committees that listen to reports of their findings, or to participate in the
design and conduct of the studies. Your ability to serve and how useful
you are to the effort will depend upon your understanding of the procedures employed.

It can be very informative to study what kinds of patients are using
your services, and to assess their special characteristics and needs. For
example, after the Korean War many of our female patients sought psychiatric help soon after having babies. After treating more than thirty of
these psychiatric maternity patients, we began a series of researches to
investigate their problems, details of which will be discussed in subsequent chapters. These investigations ultimately led to our developing
improvements in the treatment and prevention of emotional disorders of
pregnancy and childbearing (Gordon, Gordon & Gunther, 1961; Gordon,
Kapostins & Gordon, 1965). Many of the research principles described
in this book will be illustrated with studies of psychiatric maternity
patients.

To weigh the importance of new procedures. Patients' histories, signs,
symptoms, and laboratory tests are all related statistically to their diagnoses and treatment plans. New diagnostic and treatment techniques are
being developed every year. Some are expensive and time-consuming.

Do they add to the validity of a diagnosis or the effectiveness of a treatment? If you know how to find answers to these questions, you can make better decisions about whether to include them in your practice.

To practice scientific psychiatry. Insurance companies and other third-party payers are requiring that you provide quantitative evidence of the necessity for what you are doing with your patients. Since the *Diagnostic and Statistical Manual of Mental Disorders (DSM-III)* (American Psychiatric Association, 1980) introduced quantification in psychiatric diagnosis with its use of Axes IV and V to measure patients' aggravating stresses and premorbid functional levels, some insurers are beginning to ask for patient diagnoses that include all five *DSM-III* axes. Courts and juries respect the greater precision you provide when you can speak accurately about the reliability and validity of the test you used or about the objective measures of improvement in the patient you treated. This book teaches you to assess psychopathology in quantitative terms so that you can respond appropriately to the demands being made on you.

If you spend a few hours a week analyzing what you are accomplishing in your work, you can also provide yourself with morale-boosting positive feedback. By measuring your patients' characteristics before, during, and after treatment, you can determine which therapies are working with whom and which can be discarded. You can learn what you need to study in your reading and in your continuing education courses.

Furthermore, if you know how to perform needs assessments, to analyze social indicators, or to conduct program evaluations, for example, you can present data much more effectively in quality assurance committees, as an expert witness in court, or in case presentations before colleagues. This knowledge has commercial value: You can be paid well to make such analyses and presentations. Testing your patients with standardized instruments is also a reimbursable service for which you should receive payment.

Likewise, if you are called upon to conduct peer reviews of your colleagues' work, you benefit from being able to think quantitatively about it. Do the measured assessments of the patients' diagnosis, needs, and problems justify the length and cost of the treatment? Is the treatment chosen the most effective and efficient?

To improve patients' cooperation. When patients can see objective evidence of the nature of their problem, they understand the rationale of their treatment plan and can cooperate better in therapy. As you continue to assess their progress in treatment with objective measures, such as anxiety or depression inventories and measures of their improved functioning, and give them feedback on the findings, you help sustain their morale and their enthusiasm to continue in treatment with you. And when your patients know about the measured effectiveness of your efforts with previous patients who had problems and test findings similar to theirs, you can win greater cooperation from them in following your therapeutic regimen. For example, you may increase their compliance in taking medications and thus decrease their relapse rate.

To enjoy satisfactions from publishing. Publishing scientific studies can provide you with a number of additional satisfactions: fulfilling a personal need to contribute in an area of special importance to you; realizing that you are in the forefront of knowledge in a field; seeing your name and creations in print; receiving professional recognition and referrals of patients from colleagues who recognize your expertise in the field about which you have written; influencing the development of scientific psychiatry; or receiving requests from editors and publishers to write a chapter or book.

If you conduct research and evaluation projects you will expand your circle of friends to include collaborators – fellow professionals in other disciplines, graduate students, colleagues with statistical, computer, and other research expertise – with whom you ordinarily might not be working closely in your routine clinical practice. Many of these bright collaborators may become close friends whose interests broaden your horizons and enrich your life.

Some members of your family may want to become research colleagues. They may be able to help calculate statistics, write up reviews of relevant literature, and otherwise cooperate in your research studies. Of course your confidential relationship with your patients must be protected, but your collaborators never need to see a patient's chart or learn a patient's name. Most of our own studies include the names of both spouses; many also add those of one or more of our children who worked with us when they were attending high school and university.

To help discover new scientific laws. Laws state regular associations between objects and events. Laws do not have to state cause–effect relationships between phenomena; any regular relationship can be a law. You need not be a full-time researcher to describe lawful relationships. For example, the descriptions of different psychiatric diagnoses in *DSM-III* state lawful relationships among the characteristics of people given the diagnoses. But many of the psychiatrists who helped develop *DSM-III* were primarily clinicians. This book will discuss the development of some psychiatric laws.

The microcomputer and research

Microcomputers have simplified most of your research tasks. They can search the literature; assess patients directly with standardized tests; print out detailed reports; assist in monitoring patient care, reviewing utilization of treatment resources, evaluating programs, and carrying out other quality assurance procedures; perform both simple statistical and complicated multivariate and other analyses; store data and write-ups for later use; communicate with mainframe computers, colleagues, hospitals, and research files; tap databases with the help of a modem and the telephone lines; serve as word processors to write articles; print publishable tables and graphs; send your papers directly back and forth to the publisher with a modem and telephone; and even publish your reports with the help of new software. We are working on computer programs, described in chapter 8, for the microcomputer to develop quantitative treatment plans and to assist with peer review.

Computers reduce the boredom of and errors in calculating statistics by hand. Furthermore, statistical programs now available for the microcomputer are so simple and easy to run that your office secretary can plug in the data without having to understand how to do research or to calculate statistics, or even what the numbers mean. New statistical tests are being developed and new programs are being written for the personal computer each year.

As a result, the microcomputer may cause a major problem in your not too distant future: You may find yourself flooded by reports, in the literature and from staff in quality assurance, peer review, and utilization review, that are full of statistically analyzed data of dubious worth produced by microcomputers in the hands of people with greater or less understanding of what they are writing. They may spatter their texts with names to impress you – "Mann-Whitney U Test," "goodness of fit," "discriminant function analysis," "Yates's correction for continuity." You will need to wade through this scientific and pseudoscientific deluge and strain out those studies with real merit from those that are just all wet. And you will need to be able to translate the jargon and know what it means.

The chapters that follow will explain when to use various statistics and what you can do with them. They will show you how to calculate by hand the most common statistics and statistical tests – χ^2, standard deviations, t tests, phi coefficients, contingency coefficients, Spearman's rank and Pearson's product-moment correlations – those that you will need in order to conduct studies of your own patients. They will also provide examples of these statistics performed with a microcomputer.

The book will discuss the more complicated statistical tests (and those with complicated names) and explain their purposes and limitations. It will also spell out when you should seek consultation from an expert in statistics or psychiatric research. Thus it will help you to avoid and to recognize misuse of statistical programs. Finally, it will also discuss the other uses of the home and office microcomputer.

Stages of research

This book uses the following six categories or stages to classify psychiatric research (R. P. Youtz, personal communication, 1981).

1. Research to formulate an initial working hypothesis, or initial working hypothesis research
2. Research to develop measuring instruments, or measurement research
3. Observed relation research
4. Observed causal research
5. Causal relation research
6. Theory development

Science is progressive, and researchers use what has gone before. New scientific concepts generally go through most of the stages above. In the chapters that follow, you will read first of initial hypotheses about several concepts; then you will see how to measure them; later you will explore their development through observed relation, observed causal, and causal relation stages and, finally, theory development. The book will follow the development of six concepts in particular – disease and impairment, functional level, stress, social support, coping skills, and socioeconomic status – through most of the stages above.

When you read other people's studies and when you conduct your own, it is useful to determine where the research fits into this system so that you know what conclusions you can draw from the findings and what work is needed next. When you read how to perform a certain type of research, you are also learning what to look for in others' studies. Before we go further into a discussion of the stages of research, let us look at the steps you must go through in performing each research study.

Steps in conducting research

In order to conduct a publishable study, you must go through the following steps. Depending upon the type of research and your own situation, you may also want to include other procedures, such as prior consultation with other professionals or a pilot test on a few selected subjects. But the following steps are important if you intend to produce a report that will arrest the attention of your colleagues or the editors of professional journals. For the less obvious steps, we have indicated why the step is required. In chapter 3, we explain how the step is put into practice.

1. Make a hypothesis. A hypothesis is sometimes described as an educated guess about what you expect to happen under certain conditions. For example, you may have gained an impression from your clinical observations over a period of time that patients with Symptom A respond to Drug X better than to Drug Y. This can become your research hypothesis – a statement of what you believe will actually occur.

2. Read the relevant literature. Other researchers and practitioners may have noticed the same phenomena you are observing. They may already have conducted the study you are contemplating, in which case you may be wasting your time doing it over again. (Of course, you may decide that the study needs replication.) It is worse than disconcerting to spend months conducting a careful study, only to receive a reply from the editor of a publication where you submitted your report stating that this research was conducted and published by someone else years ago.

3. Decide on the type of subjects needed.

4. Decide on test instruments needed.

5. Design the study. Steps 3 and 4 start off the work of research design. Now you must decide how many patients to use and who will administer the test instruments and when.

6. Decide what statistics you will use. Make this decision before you start to collect data. Otherwise, you may amass a great deal of information that is destined to fill the back of a file drawer because there is no way to summarize it. To avoid this sad result, you must consider the statistical treatment before the data are collected.

7. Decide how many subjects you will use. In general, the rule here is the more subjects, the better. However, time, money, availability, and the law of diminishing returns will restrict the number of subjects you can use. Later chapters discuss this matter further.

8. Obtain permission to conduct research with human subjects.

9. Determine what other resources you will need. You need to consider personnel to conduct the study, administrative support, equipment, supplies, and monetary costs.

10. Make up data-collection forms. These must be standardized so that the same data will be collected from each patient in the same way.

11. Collect data. You are now ready to conduct the study. You have prepared your data-collection forms in advance and made your decisions about who will collect the data and when and where, and how the data will be analyzed. You have provided for patient confidentiality, if necessary, and made provision for the appropriate use of the data.

12. Do the arithmetic analyses. Your collected data will now fit the requirements of the statistic you chose in item 6 above, so you need only to plug the numbers into its formula. With simple directions, this work can usually be done inexpensively by your office personnel or, as in many of our studies, by your children.

13. Write up results. Chapter 4, "Research to Develop Measuring Instruments," provides details on how this should be done.

14. Choose an appropriate publication and submit your report. You should select a journal that deals with the types of topics you are studying.

15. Rework and resubmit a rejected article. Journal editors are usually generous in the amount of time and thought they spend in explaining why an article must be rejected. Heed their advice before sending your article to another journal.

Chapters 2 and 3 discuss all 15 of these steps more fully. Now we return to the stages of research and tell where they are discussed in this book.

Stages of research (continued)

1. Research to formulate an initial working hypothesis (initial working hypothesis research). The first step in conducting research is to develop a hypothesis. But generating an initial working hypothesis can itself be the first stage of research. When you get a researchable idea, you first formulate an initial working hypothesis statement. Not all the terms in the statement have yet been defined operationally, nor have their relationships to each other been demonstrated. Chapter 2 provides a number of examples of hypotheses and discusses where to submit initial working hypothesis research reports for publication. Later chapters illustrate how to follow up on many initial hypotheses, proceeding through the various stages described here.

2. Research to develop measuring instruments (measurement research). You can begin to perform measurement research when you have clearly defined your concept in words and have found or developed a specifiable physiological, chemical, physical, or psychosocial technique for assessing it. Chapter 4 discusses methods of conducting measurement research and provides examples, including standardized psychiatric rating scales. It describes the development and validation of new clinical tests for measuring patients' characteristics, and presents some studies of the clinical usefulness of *DSM-III*'s two quantitative scales, Axis IV and Axis V. Chapter 4.A shows how to calculate chi-square (χ^2), the contingency coefficient (C), the standard deviation (SD), and a t test.

3. Observed relation research. Once you have worked out how to measure two concepts, you can conduct observed relation research. This is also sometimes known as correlational research. In it you observe relationships between the two measures; you may or may not hold other factors constant.

Observed relation research may permit predictions, but it does not prove causality. Chapter 5 discusses and presents examples of observed relation research. It shows how to conduct epidemiological studies and assessments of the needs of special groups of patients such as veterans, chronic patients, and rape victims, and provides examples of the use of

DSM-III's quantitative scales in epidemiological research. It discusses where to submit these kinds of studies for publication. Chapter 5.A explains how to compute a Spearman's rank correlation, Pearson's product-moment correlation, and the unit normal variate (z).

4. Observed causal research. In many experiments in clinical treatment, you will not be able to control all factors fully. Your study may then be considered *halfway observed causal* (or sometimes *quasi-experimental*). For practical reasons many program evaluations and quality assurance studies fall into this category. Chapter 6 describes observed causal research. Examples are presented of program evaluations that extend prior needs assessments: eclectic treatment with psychiatric outpatients, geographic unitization of a veterans' psychiatric treatment program, and a psychoeducational program for chronic mental patients.

5. Causal relation research. In causal relation research you, the researcher, manipulate one of two measured variables – the independent or treatment variable. The treatment variable has at least two levels, and you hold constant all other possible conditions. You measure the changes in the dependent variable that are attributed to the treatment variable, and thus conduct fully experimental research. Chapter 7 describes causal relation research and presents examples that extend the previous work with maternity psychiatric and chronic mental patients.

6. Theory development. Many scientists rank the developing and testing of a theory as the peak of research and the most prestigious kind. A theory explains the lawful relationships that exist in the field. It describes events in such a way as to organize and classify knowledge, explain laws, and predict new laws.

A theoretical article need not present original data; however, it integrates research findings from measurement, observed relation, observed causal, and causal relation research. Theories summarize the results of other research, make generalizations based on their findings, and suggest directions for new studies. Chapter 8 discusses a theory – the functional level equation – developed from a formulation presented by Albee (1982). This theory, which is related to *DSM-III*'s multiaxial system, pulls together research described in the earlier chapters of this book. The work under way to test the theory, and its implications for the clinical practitioner, are discussed.

Research ethics

Chapter 9 discusses the important topic of research ethics. It deals with relationships with patients, research collaborators, consultants, cooperating clinicians, and fellow authors whose reports you have read or heard.

Summary

Chapter 10 reviews the themes discussed in the book, presenting them from the perspective of improving the practice of scientific psychiatry.

2. Research to formulate an initial working hypothesis

This chapter discusses hypotheses both as independent first stages of research and as one of the 15 research steps. Those of the 15 steps that are pertinent in research to formulate an initial working hypothesis are also developed more fully here. The chapter helps you prepare your own initial hypotheses for publication and describes papers that present this stage of research. It and later chapters discuss where each study was published and explain the reasons for submitting to a specific journal. Chapter 2 also includes a section on descriptive statistics for presenting information about patients in initial working hypothesis and other research reports.

Definitions

An *initial working hypothesis* is one in which not all the terms have yet been defined operationally and the relationship expressed has not been demonstrated. A hypothesis is a statement that is assumed to be true for the purpose of testing its validity (McBurney, 1983). An *operational definition* provides a statement of the precise meaning of a concept expressed in terms of an operation or procedure. Concepts like repression, cathexis, and many others commonly used in dynamic psychotherapy are very hard to define in terms of operations that any person can observe or measure. On the other hand, those like anxiety can be defined operationally in terms of a description in the American Psychiatric Association's *Diagnostic and Statistical Manual of Mental Disorders (DSM-III)* or by a score on a test for measuring anxiety or by a reading of the galvanic skin response or by pulse and breathing rates. Concepts like aggravating stress, environmental supports, and functional level have stimulated a great deal of quantitative psychiatric research because they can be defined operationally, as will be shown later.

You may content yourself with simply presenting your hypothesis in a single paper, or you may follow up by testing it in measurement, observed relation, or causal relation research. In order to perform research to formulate an initial working hypothesis, you must carry out only the following 5 of the 15 steps mentioned previously: (2) read the literature; (3) select subjects as examples; (13) write up results; (14) choose an appropriate publication and submit study; and (15) heed the editors' advice, rework, and resubmit. Many published psychiatric reports can be included in this category. Research at the initial working hypothesis stage mainly involves reading, condensing, organizing, and reporting on the literature – a process that is sometimes called *library research*. The sections that follow discuss the steps above.

Making quantifiable hypotheses

Present your hypotheses in terms that can be defined operationally in objective, quantifiable form. Then you or others can test them in quantified experiments. You arrive at new hypotheses through personal impression, experience, reading, discussion, reviewing findings from new research, or investigating a new theory. For example, while reading a scientific article you may develop a new hypothesis for explaining the research findings and may wish to report your interpretation of the events.

In addition to reporting your hypotheses separately in initial working hypothesis articles, you may present them in the *introduction* of hypothesis-testing articles that go on to describe one or more of the later stages of research in the *method, results, discussion,* and *summary* sections (see chapter 3). The discussion section of a study in which you had been testing an earlier hypothesis may also contain a new hypothesis that was generated by the results you obtained. This chapter considers the development of hypotheses both as independent types of research and as steps in the conduct of other stages of research.

Kinds of clinical hypotheses

Most clinical hypotheses are concerned with (1) the usefulness of new laboratory and other instruments or techniques for measuring patients or (2) the needs, problems, responses, and other characteristics of patients or (3) the effectiveness of new therapies.

Hypotheses with new measuring techniques or tests

New tests and instruments often pave the way for studies that investigate the biological substrate of mental disorders and other behaviors, including the anatomical, chemical, and physiological underpinnings of affective disorders, anxiety and phobias, and schizophrenia. Clinical psychiatrists who gain access to new tests and laboratory instruments can study their usefulness with their office and hospital patients.

For example, an electroencephalogram provided a tool for testing a hypothesis about relationships between biomedical characteristics – abnormal brainwaves – and performance – success or failure in nursing school (R. E. Gordon, Kapostins & Gordon, 1960).

When chemical autoanalyzers became available for performing large numbers of blood serum tests cheaply, we could explore relationships between behavior – performance in college – and two biochemicals related to disease: serum uric acid and cholesterol. These hypotheses stated that higher levels of these two chemicals were related positively to college students' academic achievement (Lindeman, Gordon & Gordon, 1969).

Hypotheses that automated multiphasic health testing might speed up and improve the reliability and validity of the clinical evaluation of patients' medical impairments led to the establishment of such a laboratory at a university health center (Clark & Gordon, 1970; R. E. Gordon, 1971; R. E. Gordon, Bielen & Watts, 1973; R. E. Gordon, Holzer, Bielen, Watts & Gordon, 1973; R. E. Gordon, Warheit, Hursch, Schwab, Watts & Gordon, 1975).

The *Diagnostic and Statistical Manual of Mental Disorders (DSM-III)* introduced and defined two new quantitative measures, Axis IV (aggravating stress) and Axis V (premorbid functional level). *DSM-III* provided data about the reliability of these scales, but suggested that researchers investigate their validity and usefulness in psychiatry.

In a theoretical article on the functional level equation we hypothesized that Axis IV, Axis V, and their ratio, the strain ratio, would be correlated with the amount of treatment that psychiatric patients need (R. E. Gordon, Jardiolin & Gordon, 1985; R. E. Gordon, Vijay, Sloate, Burket & Gordon, 1985).

You may wish to hypothesize about relationships between patient diagnoses and findings with new laboratory devices to which you gain access, equipment such as brain imaging technologies – computer axial tomography scanners, magnetic resonance imagers, positron emission tomographs. You can then explore what these instruments show with your patients. If these new tests and instruments provide better methods of assessing patients' characteristics, you may win some renown as an expert in the use of the new equipment.

Hypotheses about patients' characteristics

You may hypothesize about and report on the patients you see and the problems they encounter. We published hypotheses about the special characteristics and needs of various groups of our patients – students (R. E. Gordon, Lindeman & Gordon, 1967), private outpatients (R. E. Gordon, Gordon, Plutzky & Guerra, in press), veterans (R. E. Gordon, Warheit et al., 1975; R. E. Gordon, Bielen & Watts, 1973), and chronically ill patients in state mental hospitals (R. E. Gordon, Patterson, Eberly & Penner, 1980). These led to quantitative studies of the patients' specific needs. Sometimes you may wake up at night with the beginnings of an idea about a special feature of your patients. If so, do not ignore it or lose sleep lying in bed stewing about it. Keep a pad at your night table and put down a few notes to help you recall it in the morning. Then go back to sleep knowing you can pursue the theme at your leisure during the daytime.

Research to formulate an initial working hypothesis with psychiatric maternity patients

In the mid 1950s a very large percentage of female psychiatric patients had developed emotional disorders of pregnancy and childbearing. Clinical observations and a review of the literature led to the publication of an initial working hypothesis. It proposed that many maternity psychiatric patients were becoming distressed as a result of encountering stresses in adapting to a new role in life to which they had been negatively sensitized and with which they were poorly prepared to cope. A hypothesis could have been made that the psychiatric maternity patients were experiencing unconscious conflicts related to maternity. But how can you operationally define and objectively quantify the dynamic unconscious? Because this kind of concept prevailed in the thinking of that period, few studies had attempted to quantify the stresses and other psychosocial factors in psychiatric patients' lives.

As is shown in later chapters, the initial hypothesis above about psychiatric maternity patients led to a sequence of increasingly higher stages of research with childbearing women. Likewise, many initial working hypotheses mentioned in this chapter were made in the expectation that later research would use them in quantitative experiments.

Do not hesitate to modify your hypothesis if the data point to a need to do so. Analyses of quantitative data from the maternity psychiatric studies revealed that a high percentage of these women were undergoing stresses associated with their being newcomers to the community, having recently moved from another county or state. A maternity questionnaire (see chapter 4) assessed these stresses in a series of studies. A factor analysis (see chapter 5) of the data from these studies led to a new hypothesis, namely, that the psychiatric maternity patients' problems were associated in part with an accumulation of stresses – background sensitizers in their lives, such as the death of a parent or a severe personal illness, and present-day pressurizers such as their assuming the new maternal role, moving to a new home, and taking on other burdens related to social mobility without adequate social support.

The research on relationships between social mobility and psychiatric disorder among maternity patients led to an expanded hypothesis that stresses from social mobility were important in the illnesses of many other patients of both sexes and all ages. Studies of patients' characteristics and needs frequently lead to hypotheses about new therapies that might help them better cope with their problems.

Hypotheses about new therapies

You may want to try out a new medication or other kind of therapy in your office or hospital. During the early 1950s psychoactive drugs and social learning therapy were first becoming available in psychiatry. We hypothesized that treatment that combined psychotropic medications, behavior management, training in social skills and supports, and dynamic therapy, as needed, would improve patients' functioning better than would each different kind of treatment given separately (R. E. Gordon, Singer & Gordon, 1961).

Later, concern about the practice of polypharmacy with psychoactive drugs led to the hypothesis that a self-medication system involving a single bedtime dose could use psychoeducational and behavior management methods to teach chronic mental patients to medicate themselves properly (Cohen, Gordon, Adams, Marlowe, Bedell & Weathers, 1979).

Reading the relevant literature

In the field of psychiatry, where patient variables are many and complex and quantitative research is relatively new, you are likely to find that reviewing the literature is well worth your time. You may discover that someone else has already done the work you are planning. Even more likely is the possibility that your literature search will disclose that others have taken a different approach to your research question. They may have used a different age or population group or a different method of looking at patient responses that may be relevant to your study. Often you will find that the published research to date is related to the problem you intend to attack but that there are some important differences between others' work and your ideas. For example, a literature review of stress and serum chemical levels turned up articles about medical students, college professors, and high school students, but none about football players. This is the best possible situation for you if you are interested in studying the last group. It means that you will want to refer to the work when offering your completed study for publication but will point out exactly how it differs from yours and possibly how and why the results are different.

When other studies appear in the literature regarding the same or a similar problem (either the same patient qualities or the same treatments), you know that the profession is interested in and concerned with that group or that treatment. Your work, then, is current and of vital interest to your colleagues. You may even have found the key to the entire problem. This makes your work highly important and publishable.

These are the main reasons for a careful look at the literature before you start. Others may surface as you read the articles; for instance, you may decide to contact other researchers to find out more about their studies than the published work reveals. Or you may find that a practitioner in your geographic area is working on the same question; you might want to join forces with him or her. But at the very least, a careful perusal of the literature is necessary to keep you from reinventing the wheel and to enhance the scope and relevance of your research.

MEDLARS and MEDLINE

Computers now make the task of reviewing the literature quite simple. MEDLARS, the Medical Literature Analysis and Retrieval System of the National Library of Medicine in Bethesda, Maryland, provides a number of databases in an online network. Of most importance to you is the MEDLINE, which in 1983 contained more than 800,000 references to biomedical journal articles published in that and the three preceding years. At that time, 1,902 centers in locations all over the United States had access to MEDLINE. Table 2.1 presents an excerpt from a MEDLINE report of articles on postpartum psychosis that appeared during the years 1982 through 1985.

Your hospital library can contact a center in your area and obtain the literature search you request. If you have a microcomputer and a modem, you can gain access to the MEDLINE file yourself over the telephone

Table 2.1. *A MEDLINE report on publications on postpartum psychosis (AU = author; TI = title; SO = source)*

```
1
AU  - De Leo D ; Galligioni S ; Magni G
TI  - A case of Capgras delusion presenting as a postpartum psychosis.
SO  - J Clin Psychiatry 1985 Jun;46(6):242-3

2
AU  - Munoz RA
TI  - Postpartum psychosis as a discrete entity.
SO  - J Clin Psychiatry 1985 May;46(5):182-4

3
AU  - Riley DM ; Watt DC
TI  - Hypercalcemia in the etiology of puerperal psychosis.
SO  - Biol Psychiatry 1985 May;20(5):479-88

4
AU  - Hurt LD ; Ray CP
TI  - Postpartum disorders. Mother-infant bonding on a psychiatric
      unit.
SO  - J Psychosoc Nurs Ment Health Serv 1985 Feb;23(2):15-20

5
AU  - Kendell RE
TI  - Emotional and physical factors in the genesis of puerperal mental
      disorders.
SO  - J Psychosom Res 1985;29(1):3-11

6
AU  - Matheson I ; Evang A ; Over: KF ; Syversen G
TI  - Presence of chlorprothixene and its metabolites in breast milk.
SO  - Eur J Clin Pharmacol 1984;27(5):611-3

7
AU  - Arizmendi TG ; Affonso DD
TI  - Research on psychosocial factors and postpartum depression: a
      critique.
SO  - Birth 1984 Winter;11(4):237-45
```

lines. MEDLINE covers articles from 3,000 journals published in the United States and foreign countries. It provides an English abstract, if one is included in the article. You can search online (or ask a medical librarian to search for you) periods back to 1966 on backfiles that total 3,500,000 references. In addition to MEDLINE, MEDLARS provides databases on toxicology, cancer, ethics, and twelve other subjects of interest to medical researchers.

Deciding on the type of subjects you will need

Initial working hypothesis studies frequently report case histories that illustrate the theme of the report. These usually describe patients seen in the author's clinical practice. If you intend to include case histories in a paper, you must obtain the permission of the patients whose examples you chose. You must also disguise the stories by using initials or changing names and by omitting all irrelevant identifying details that might infringe upon the privacy of the patients (see chapter 9).

You may also wish to describe the characteristics of groups of patients you have seen that led to your developing your hypotheses. Descriptive statistics help you perform this task.

The arithmetic of descriptive statistics

You may have, or may be able to obtain, large batches of patient data, such as an accumulation of data about Vietnam veterans or disaster victims seeking psychiatric help in your area, that are interesting in and of themselves. If you feel that a description of the characteristics of these patients would interest your colleagues, you need a method for describing what you have found without listing each record individually.

The field of *descriptive statistics* supplies you with methods for succinctly describing the interesting facts to your colleagues. Besides providing convenient summary statements, these statistics may also be used later to make comparisons between this set of data and some other set that you may obtain from your own practice or that someone else may obtain from some other source. The following descriptive statistics are used to summarize data.

The range

The range of a variable is its extent. For example, to obtain the range of ages of your Vietnam patients, you run through the entire batch, tabulating ages as you go, and then pick out the youngest and the oldest cases. You will now be able to state, for example: The ages range from 31.5 years to 45.5 years.

You may also want to investigate the length of time each of these men spent in the service, in this country or in Vietnam or both. Again, you will tabulate their service times and state the range: from 1 year to 4.5 years total service time, or from 1 to 3.8 years overseas.

You may consider it interesting to know how evenly the cases are spread over these ranges. For example, are most of the veterans closer to 31.5 years or to the upper end of the scale? Or do they group together somewhere in the middle? The range will not give you an answer. You may have 350 cases between 31.5 and 38, then 47 between ages 38 and 40, and only 3 over age 40. You need a statement that will summarize this distribution of ages – a *measure of central tendency.*

Measures of central tendency: mean, median, and mode

When you have a large amount of data, you generally want to find out what the "usual" case is like. Such information will lead you to develop ideas and hypotheses about the patient group you are interested in. The few unusual cases may be interesting in their own right as case studies, but they may not give you much useful information about the more common cases or about the group as a whole.

There are several measures of central tendency that you can use, depending upon (1) what kind of data you have, (2) what kinds of statements you want to make about the data, and (3) what further use you intend to make of the data. It is necessary to understand the following points about central tendency and variability because they determine the kinds of statistics – parametric or nonparametric – that you can use to analyze your data. (The meanings of the terms *parametric* and *nonparametric* will be discussed in the chapters that follow.)

The mean. The most commonly used measure of central tendency is the arithmetic mean. This is the common average, which you use to compute your grade-point average in college, your average telephone bill, or any other amount where you want the usual figure uncomplicated by incidental aberrations. It is the sum of the values of all the cases divided by the number of cases. This is represented by the simple formula

Mean = sum of the values of the variable/total number of cases

Applying this formula to your veterans, you may come out with a figure of 34.32 years, which is the mean age of Vietnam veterans receiving treatment. There may be no individual veteran whose age is 34.32 years. This is simply the arithmetic mean of all your veterans' ages.

Note also that this figure is not necessarily at the middle of the range. It is closer to the lower end of the range than it is to the upper end. When the mean is nearer one end of the range than the other, you can usually assume that there are more cases near that end than the other. However, it is also true that a few unusual cases at one end of the range of a distribution can pull the mean in their direction. A well-known example of this lies in the averaging of incomes in a community: There may be many people in the lower income range, say around $15,000 a year, but including just a few people who earn $250,000 a year will skew the mean upward so that the resulting figure will give the impression that the whole community consists of people with higher than average incomes. In like manner, if a few of your Vietnam veterans happened to be aged 76 (highly unlikely), the mean age of the group would be pulled up toward the high end of the range.

A rule to remember, then, in dealing with means is: The mean can be skewed by a few unusual cases at one end of a wide range. However, the more cases you have, the less the mean will be skewed in either direction by the unusual cases.

The mean is the most useful measure of central tendency for comparing one batch of data with some other batch. It is used in many high-powered parametric statistics by which you compare the mean of one group with that of another for the variables you are measuring. This is not true of the next two measures of central tendency, but there is much useful information to be gained from them.

The median. You might want to know where the midpoint of the range is so that you can talk about the upper half and the lower half. This would also reduce the influence of a few unusual cases. A meaningful statistic, then, would be one that divided the cases in half. The statistic for this is the median. For example, with the salary range from zero to $250,000, you may find that 200 of the veterans earn less than $26,500 per year, while the other half earn over $26,500 per year. Therefore,

Median = the point on the range below which 50% of the cases
fall and above which the other 50% fall

Again, as with the mean, there may be no case at all that falls on the median itself; there may be no veteran earning exactly $26,500 per year. Also, the range may extend much farther on one side of the median than on the other; or, in statistical terms, the distribution is skewed. But the value of the median would not be affected by a very successful veteran's earning $250,000 per year, whereas the mean certainly would be. If, instead, the highest salary were $65,900 per year, the median would still be at $26,500.

There are a number of nonparametric tests that make use of the median, such as the Kruskal–Wallis one-way analysis of variance (see chapters 3 and 4).

The mode. You still may ask, "Where do *most* of the cases fall?" The two measures of central tendency above tell you a great deal about age and income. What about time in service? Here you have a short range – from 1 year to 4.5 years. You want to know how much time most of the men spent in service. For this question, we use the mode. This is the number where the highest frequency falls. To compute it, you first divide service time into some convenient numbers like months (you can make this scale very rough, using only whole years, or very fine, using numbers of days). Then we have a scale going from 12 months to 54 months.

Make a check mark for each veteran under the number of months served. Usually, one month will have more check marks than any other. For example, suppose you find that under 36 months you have 175 cases and that all the other months have fewer than 175 check marks. Then 36 months is the mode for your distribution of months in service.

Mode = the value with the highest frequency

Sometimes you will find that there are two values with equally high frequencies. In that case, your distribution is said to be *bimodal.* There could be any number of modes. If there is more than one, it is usually a good idea to collapse your measure (from single months to three-month periods, for example) and thus rearrange your data so that there is no more than one mode.

There are many interesting statistical properties of bimodal distributions, but most of them are beyond the scope of this book. Suffice it to say that if you intend to make comparisons of your set of data with some other, it will be to your advantage to work with data having only one mode. When you find that you have more than one mode on a variable of interest, it may mean (1) that you have cut your variable too fine. That is, if we tabulated length of service in terms of days served and had only 400 cases, there might very well be two or three more modal values. But if we tabulated in terms of half-years, there would very likely be only one mode. Or (2) – a possibility with more serious implications – it could be that you really have samples from two different populations.

For example, a study of migratory disabled veterans admitted to the psychiatric service of a Veterans Administration hospital (Gordon, Lyons, Muniz & Most, 1973) found that the overall mean for the total sample of 86 men was 39 years, but there was a bimodal distribution. The mean age for 35 patients was 26 years, and for 51 it was 49 years. These two groups represented different populations; one group consisted of World War II and Korean War veterans and the other of

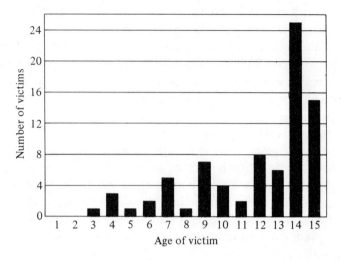

Figure 2.1. A bar graph showing the age distribution of child rapes in Denver for 1973.
(From Hursch, 1977, fig. 2, p. 27.)

Vietnam veterans. Since these might represent patients with two very different kinds of problems, we may not have wanted to mix the data from these two groups of veterans.

Unlike the mean and the median, the mode will always have many cases falling on the exact modal value. It is the only one of the three measures of central tendency with this characteristic.

The most common use of the mode is the graphical representation of data in a histogram (bar graph), where the frequency distribution of the values of a variable is shown by means of rectangles whose widths represent class intervals and whose heights represent corresponding frequencies. This is the familiar, easily understood graph that is used in many different forms in newspapers and magazines. When the frequency distribution of one variable is depicted, the highest bar in the graph is the mode. Figure 2.1 presents an example of a bar graph with the mode at 14 years.

Frequency distribution

This is the tabulation of the number of cases occurring at each value of a given variable. It is used in the calculation of many statistics. Examples of frequency distributions appear in Tables 4.2, 5.6, 7.4, 7.5, and 8.7.

Measures of variability

After you have computed whichever measure of central tendency will work best for your purposes, you will want to know how wide the spread is around the "middle" measure. The range tells you only the outer limits of the variable. You do not know how the cases are grouped within the range; they may be clustered closely around the mean or be a long way from it or both.

Standard deviation. The standard deviation is a measure that tells how the scores differ from the mean. It is based upon the difference (plus or minus) between each individual case and the group mean. It is defined as:

> Standard deviation = the square root of: the sum of each squared deviation from the mean/number of cases minus 1, or $SD = \sqrt{\Sigma Dev^2/(N-1)}$

(Calculation of the standard deviation is discussed more fully in chapter 4.A.) The square of the standard deviation is called the *variance,* an important statistic in measuring variability of a collection of data. For an explanation of the logic underlying the quantities represented in the equation for the standard deviation and the variance, we refer the interested reader to Runyon's *Fundamentals of Statistics in the Biological, Medical, and Health Sciences* (1985). The squaring procedure allows the formula to take account of differences both above and below the mean without having them cancel each other out. "Number of cases minus 1" represents a quantity called *degrees of freedom,* which is discussed briefly in chapter 4.A and explained more fully in most statistics textbooks, including those mentioned in chapter 5.A.

There are many uses of the standard deviation and the variance (see chapters 3, 4, and 5).

The normal curve

The normal curve is the basis for many statistics. It is the familiar bell-shaped curve, with a high mound in the middle and ends that gradually slope downward and out to infinity (see Figure 2.2). We are concerned with some of its properties:

1. Distribution. Stating that a trait is normally distributed means that if we measured it for everybody in the population (or for a very large num-

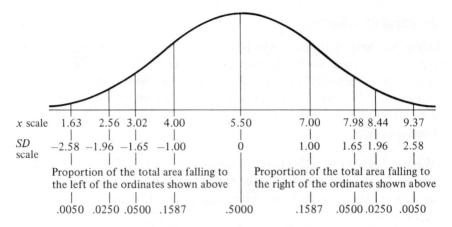

Figure 2.2. The normal curve. In this example the mean of the *x* values equals 5.5, and the standard deviation (*SD*) of the *x* values equals 1.5.

The unit normal variate, *z* (discussed in chapter 5), standardizes scores so that the probability of their occurrence can be related to the area under this curve. Table A.4 in the Appendix lists the probability of each value of *z*.

ber of cases), a line drawn over the values of its frequency distribution would look very much like the normal curve. When this is true, we can make use of all the known properties of the normal curve to form our conclusions about that trait in the population.

2. Symmetry. The curve is the same shape to the right of the midline as to the left of the midline. This means that the distribution is not skewed toward either end of the scale.

3. Central tendency. On the ideal normal curve shown in Figure 2.2, the mean, median, and mode all have the same value, and this value occurs in the exact middle of the distribution. There are also the same number of values at both ends of the distribution.

4. Deviations from the mean. If we extended a line representing the value of the standard deviation of a trait out from the mean toward one end of the curve, and then drew a straight line down to the baseline, we would find that exactly 34% of the population fell in the area between this line and one from the mean of the curve to the baseline. Therefore, at the mean plus and minus one standard deviation, we would include 68% of the population. At the mean plus and minus two standard deviations, we would include 95% of the population (thus the familiar statement expressed in scientific presentations, "the value is within two standard deviations from the mean"), and at plus or minus three standard deviations, we would include 99+% of the population.

These properties of the normal curve make it possible for us to make inferences from the sample we have tested to the general population – including all the people we did not test – on the trait we are measuring, if we have good reason to believe that the trait is normally distributed in the population.

Writing up results – a few tips on style

Many good books address this topic quite fully. However, a few suggestions will help the inexperienced writer gain the favorable attention of editors and reviewers. First, look at the style and format of articles in several issues of the journal where you plan to submit. Try to write in the same manner. Whenever possible, use simple declarative sentences and choose action verbs. Most readers, physicians included, feel most comfortable when reading at least two levels below their top reading grade level.

There is nothing wrong with using the first person plural ("We found ... ") when you have worked with and discussed your ideas with a colleague on a research project. (The *American Journal of Psychiatry,* however, wants you to use the third person.) Try to write short sentences, explaining concepts in simple English as if to a layman. Avoid passive, weak constructions like "It is believed that ... " Use headings and subheadings that help the reader focus on the topic you are discussing.

Choosing an appropriate publication and submitting the article

There is some standardization among journals in the same field regarding the format of articles submitted, but there are many specialized journals with particular requirements. These cover such details as desired number of pages, method of citing references, use of footnotes, and other technicalities. Journals frequently print these in several issues during the year. If not, write to the editor while your work is still in progress for a copy of the list of requirements.

You should think about what you are seeking to accomplish in writing your article and aim it at an audience who is interested in its thesis. Try to select a title that tells your readers what to expect in the article and that draws their attention to it. The following paragraphs describe some of the characteristics of various publications where you may submit your papers.

District branch (DB) newsletters. Here you can discuss your ideas on clinical, political, and economic issues of interest to your psychiatric colleagues. DB newsletter editors are usually looking for material, so you can get a well-written report into print in a short time without going through the lengthy process of critical review by independent referees. If you want to establish your priority with a new hypothesis or keep your copyright, you may want to publish in your DB's newsletter (Alderman, Gordon, Gordon, Ahsanuddin & Slaymaker, 1984).

Articles in psychiatric newsletters also serve a political purpose. They inform your colleagues of your special areas of interest and ability. They may help get you referrals, but more likely may result in your getting appointed to a committee or elected to an office in your district branch. Many successful leaders in the American Psychiatric Association have used their district branch newsletters to help them rise to the fore politically.

State medical journals. Articles in state medical journals inform your nonpsychiatric medical colleagues about clinical matters that interest them and that they do not have time to review on their own. If well received, they can help build your clinical practice and win the respect of colleagues in your state. Editors and readers of state medical society journals look favorably upon well-written articles that present new clinical hypotheses, contain good reviews of the literature, and address clinical topics of general medical interest, whether or not they contain measurement, observed relation, or causal relation data. Review papers submitted to the state medical journal may make lead articles because they present novel ideas that appeal to the interests of the journal editors and referees. Many may lead to referrals from colleagues whose patients have the problem discussed in the article. Generally, state medical journals use referees to help screen and edit articles, so acceptance is more difficult than in the DB newsletter, and the time between submission and publication is longer.

Proprietary journals. Many pharmaceutical houses and hospital chains publish or support the publication of nonrefereed journals that promote the medications or hospital services they provide. You receive some of these journals free of charge each month. Generally they do not seek unsolicited submissions. Once you are considered an expert on a subject, one or more of them may ask you to submit an article on a topic of their choosing. Our publication of articles and books on the benefits of combined therapy led to reports for proprietary journals. Articles in proprietary journals present updates on a clinical subject addressed to all physicians rather than just to the psychiatric specialist. They are written in nontechnical style, usually without references. Proprietary journals may provide you with a token payment for your efforts, but publication in proprietary journals probably benefits you most by calling attention to your expertise and attracting referrals.

Specialty journals. Specialty journals accept initial hypothesis articles on new-frontier subjects, like "Psychiatric Screening Through Multiphasic Health Testing" (R. E. Gordon, 1971) and "Castration for Sex Offenders – Treatment or Punishment" (Heim & Hursch, 1979). Articles that emphasize new and original findings from measurement, observed relation, or causal relation data are suitable for readers of specialty journals who are interested in the scientific frontiers of their field. Later chapters of this book present titles and data from some of these articles to illustrate the points made.

Major national and international journals. Major journals like the *Journal of the American Medical Association* take articles of general international medical interest. They want a good review of the literature and convincing data in support of an observed or causal relation, as in a report entitled "Psychosomatic Problems of a Rapidly Growing Suburb," which presented observed relation data in support of a hypothesis that higher incidences of psychosomatic disorders occurred in rapidly growing communities (R. E. Gordon & Gordon, 1959). However, they also take initial hypothesis papers on fresh subjects that might interest many readers, such as a medical anthropological paper on folk healers and modern medicine (K. K. Gordon & Gordon, 1964).

Book chapters. Once again, when you are looked upon as an expert in a subject, you may receive an invitation to write a chapter for a textbook or other learned tome. Usually medical college faculty are the persons who receive this kind of invitation. Book chapters provide a thorough review of the subject, a comprehensive list of references, and original research (Edmunson, Bedell, Archer & Gordon, 1982; Edmunson, Bedell & Gordon, 1984; Hursch, 1970; Slater, Gordon & Gordon, 1978).

Resubmitting a rejected article

Do not be dismayed when your papers are returned by journal editors with "Thanks, but no thanks" letters. When they return your article, journal editors generally include detailed excerpts from the reviewers' critiques, which explain why your paper was not accepted in its present form. Pay attention to the referees' comments, many of which are very thoughtful and useful, and modify your papers carefully.

If their reason for rejecting your paper is lack of clarity of your exposition, then rewriting may result in acceptance of the article. Sometimes the rejection is due to subject matter being not right for the journal you selected. If so, try another journal where your work will more closely match the editorial needs or interests. Usually if the work has been conducted with care and your results shed light on a subject of interest to some group, you will find a journal interested in publishing it if you persist.

The paper called "Psychosomatic Problems of a Rapidly Growing Suburb" is a case in point. It went first to a specialty journal, which rejected it. Realizing that the subject matter of the study was more interesting to physicians of all specialties, we reworked it and resubmitted the report to the *Journal of the American Medical Association*. The editors there accepted it in a few weeks. When they published it, they made the paper the journal's lead article.

Summary

This chapter has looked at research to formulate an initial working hypothesis. It has considered such topics as getting research ideas from patients, from reading, from using new laboratory tests and other instruments, or from learning about new therapies. It discussed *DSM-III*'s introducing the concepts of aggravating stress and functional level and presenting two new scales – Axis IV and Axis V – to use in measuring them. The chapter mentioned hypotheses about the validity and usefulness of Axes IV and V.

Chapter 2 has also explained in detail 5 of the 15 steps necessary for setting up, executing, and publishing the results of a research study. The normal curve and descriptive statistics used in over 42% of psychiatric articles in the most important psychiatric journals (Hokanson et al., 1986) were discussed. The chapter concluded by considering where to submit an article for publication and included a few pointers on style.

Caveat

Initial working hypotheses may seem reasonable and, after publication, may receive endorsement from influential colleagues, powerful politicians, and the public. But public acceptance does not mean that fact will support a hypothesis. Unfortunately, political decisions are often made and enormous amounts of money and human energy are poured into an effort because its hypothesis is appealing. Hypotheses need to be followed up by quantitative correlational and experimental studies in the manner shown in subsequent chapters of this book before they can be accepted as valid.

3. Further steps needed in conducting research

This chapter discusses more fully the remaining steps you must take in conducting full-scale experimental research. It also explains the format you use for reporting a quantitative research study in the scientific literature or in an oral report. The chapter looks at studies you can perform both with your own patients and also with special equipment or groups of subjects to which you may have access.

The null hypothesis

In order to make a statistical test of a research hypothesis, it is necessary to state the hypothesis in a testable form. This is the *null hypothesis* that you have read about in psychiatric journals – the hypothesis upon which all statistical analyses are based. While at first glance this may seem to be a strange way to do the business of research, a moment's consideration will explain the logic involved.

Our work at a university provided us with access to a college football team who underwent complete physical and laboratory examinations in the spring and fall of each year. In the literature we had noted that the serum cholesterol (SC) and uric acid (SUA) levels of some persons were reported to rise when they were under stress (Brooks & Mueller, 1966; Kasl, Brooks & Cobb, 1966; Lindeman, Gordon & Gordon, 1969). We hypothesized: "Football players' SC and SUA levels will increase during the competitive fall football season, when the team is under greater pressure to perform, as compared to the spring of the year."

The null hypothesis for this study would be "Football players' levels of serum cholesterol and serum uric acid are the same in the fall football season as at other times of the year." There are two important factors to keep in mind:

(1) Since you already believe that SC and SUA will rise in this group, you are biased (perhaps rightly so, but you still need to prove it). The

statement that there is no difference (that is, the null hypothesis) sets up a neutral situation to eliminate any biases.

(2) Since no two human beings are likely to respond in exactly the same way to anything, your research hypothesis does not provide any way for you to come to a conclusion about how much of a difference makes a difference. If you conduct research to show that one treatment is better than another, then you will be caught in the nagging – and unanswerable – questions "How much better than?" and "Enough better to make a difference?"

On the other hand, if you start from the neutral standpoint of no difference between the responses produced by the two treatments and then do the testing carefully, you can apply statistics to the results. These will tell you not only whether or not there is a difference, but also whether or not this is a significant difference between the responses produced by the two treatments. A *significant difference* is a meaningful mathematical statement that is immediately comprehended by other researchers. Your work then has credence. Obviously your previous statement that one treatment is better than another is a subjective opinion that may be open to question and argument by all, and that may not be testable by any recognized statistical treatment.

Therefore, while your research hypothesis is what you genuinely believe, it can only be tested by restating it in the form of a null hypothesis so a statistical test can be applied to it.

Decide on the type of subjects needed

Types of subjects are discussed here. How these subjects are selected will be discussed later. Two related statistical concepts should be kept in mind when you choose your subject group – the *population* and the *sample*.

Population

Obviously, if your research findings apply only to the small group of people in your study, they are of little use to anyone else. To be of working interest to your colleagues, they must apply to a larger group of people called a *population*.

Sample

You usually do not study every member of a population. Therefore you will select a *sample* on which to do your research. At the same time, by the use of the appropriate statistics, your results should be generalizable from the sample to the rest of the population – just as the national television networks on election day select and interview a sample of voters and then accurately generalize the voting pattern to a whole district.

The makeup of your sample determines the population to which your results can be applied. For example, if your subjects are 20 young women between the ages of 23 and 25, of Swedish extraction, unmarried, each with a birthmark on her left thigh, then that is the population to whom your work is applicable. Your findings will say nothing about men of age 40 of Irish descent with or without such a birthmark. If characteristics are not essential to your study, you should not burden your results with them and thereby restrict the applicability of your work. This is one side of the coin.

The other side of the coin is that if you do not restrict some of the characteristics of your sample, your results may consistently show no difference between one treatment and the next. Suppose you tried to use the following subjects in a special study of the effects of the stress of the football season:

a 35-year-old unemployed male Vietnam veteran; a 16-year-old female with a drug problem; a semiliterate female of 35 with four young children; an upper-class society matron of 59 with hypertension; a highly manic male executive in his late 40s with a stomach ulcer; a male high school dropout, aged 17, arrested for burglary; a severely depressed 32-year-old male surgeon, recently divorced; a male homosexual, aged 35, with AIDS; a single female secretary, aged 19, who is pregnant; a retired male bank teller, aged 70, with impotence problems.

Can you imagine how confusing the serum chemical level findings might be (let alone the task of carrying out the research) if you tried to do a study of the effects of football season stress on this sample? Yet we have seen funded studies that compared the effects of two or more antidepressant drugs upon samples almost as diverse. Males and females; adolescents, adults, and the elderly; and patients with schizophrenia, organic mental disorder, alcoholism, drug addiction, and both psychotic and neurotic depression were thrown together haphazardly in each study group. These groups are so diverse that, unless the treatment really is a panacea for all human ills, like penicillin, the research has a high probability of coming up with no difference between Treatment X and Treatment Y. This is because psychiatric variables often influence and are influenced by demographic, age, sociological, diagnostic, and other variables. These unplanned influences are called *extraneous variables*. They are not your research variables, but they may affect your research variables in a wide variety of unknown ways. (In research, the term *variable* refers to some aspect of a test condition that has been measured and that can change or take on different characteristics with different conditions.)

(You will often run across the word *treatment* in research and statistical usage. In these contexts it is used in a generic or statistical sense to mean any experimental intervention. Thus it may refer to bestowing blandishments on a child for making appropriate responses, basing the rewards to teenagers on the accomplishment of required tasks, providing patients with an experimental drug, or any other procedure used in the expectation of achieving a desired effect.)

If you fail to consider extraneous variables in selecting your subjects, the wide differences among your subjects may completely obscure important differences in your treatments. The message here is: Do not needlessly restrict the range of the population to which your results might apply (as in the example of the Swedish women), and do not select a sample that represents such a diverse population that your treatment effects will be obscured by the differences among subjects.

A reasonable sample to represent the population of interest in our research was:
> A football team of young white males, between the ages of 18 and 23, all of whom are representing the same college in intercollegiate sports.

This population includes a number of people in American society who are of interest to many of our colleagues – but note that it does not include everybody. It does not include black players, because at the time of the study there were few blacks on the team in question. College football coaches sometimes develop heart attacks during the highly competitive football season, but our findings cannot be applied directly to them either.

You may have other criteria for selecting your subjects, such as diagnosis, intelligence level, a specified educational level, marital status, health record, or a specific psychiatric history like a record of previous hospitalization. In the serum chemical studies, we found that college class, age, grades, major course of study, and other variables were also correlated with serum chemical levels (see chapter 5). It was useful to look at these factors as well as the football players' positions on the team – offense, defense, running back, end, etc. – in studying their serum chemical responses to the football season.

Sometimes a group of people may be examined as a whole where the individuals are not sampled randomly. This may be the only way to conduct the research within reasonable economic or practical limits. Whereas this does not constitute random sampling of the members of the group, and therefore inferences about the results should be made with that shortcoming in mind, much useful information can be gained from such studies.

In the football players' study, the serum cholesterol levels of the players referred to above was examined for each player, but all players were on the same college team. This does not represent a random sample of all football players. To obtain a truly random sample would have necessitated putting the names of all college football players in one big drum and selecting a prespecified number of these names. However, the many differences among the diets, training, geographical influences, and other factors characteristic of these players might have obscured the serum cholesterol differences. Therefore, the latter procedure would not necessarily have resulted in a better, that is, more meaningful, study, because it would have brought in too many uncontrolled variables that could affect the results.

As the study was conducted, most of these extraneous factors were controlled naturally. For example, because the players were all on the same team, their diets were nearly identical, outside temperature and humidity conditions were the same for all, and their training was the same. It may reasonably be assumed that the players – coming from different backgrounds and geographic areas – are a self-selected random sample of college football players nationwide. At the same time, it should be kept in mind that, since the sample was a unified group at one college, the results might or might not be generalizable to other teams on other diets in other locations. As it was, the study brought to light important information that could easily be checked out on other teams.

Studies of your own patients

The same principle applies when you study a group consisting solely of your own patients. Consider it a random sample of your patients. Unless you are engaged in a special treatment practiced by no one else, it can be assumed that these people randomly selected themselves to be your patients in the first place. Strictly speaking, results may be generalized only to your own patients. However, strikingly significant results, such as those with psychiatric maternity patients (discussed previously and later in this book) and in the use of current functional level with the Axis V scale of the *Diagnostic and Statistical Manual (DSM-III)* to measure patients' progress (see chapter 4.A and chapter 8), may very well be applicable to similar patients everywhere. Such studies need to be tested and confirmed in other settings.

Few research endeavors will apply equally well to both sexes, to all ages, to every diagnosis, and to all sociological, economic, and ethnic groups. Even if the treatment you propose to research offers broad hope to humanity, you should begin your testing of that hypothesis by trying it out on specific groups first and then gradually enlarging your scope until you have included many specific groups and can justify testing it on the diverse crowd in the example above. This was the approach we took. We applied our new psychiatric treatment techniques first to psychiatric maternity patients. Next we performed a carefully controlled study of antenatal women. Then we expanded the work to include other young married women and finally a wide range of psychiatric outpatients and, still later, inpatients, as discussed in the chapters that follow.

Consider now the pros and cons of retrospectively studying data you already have collected in patients' case histories as part of their care and treatment versus starting up a prospective research program.

Retrospective and prospective studies

You have gotten a hunch in your practice, from your reading, or from some previous research you have done about what you expect to happen under certain conditions, and have made a hypothesis about it. Or you have conceived a theory that generates a number of new hypotheses. Now you must determine how you can put your hypothesis to the test. Often-times you may find it easy to examine records of patients who have been treated by you or your hospital. If this retrospective study of data that are already collected confirms your hypothesis, it will be worth while to design a prospective study. In prospective studies you carry out all 15 of the steps discussed in this chapter. But in reviewing records retrospec-tively you had no control over who the subjects were or how the data were initially recorded and collected; many important research steps may have been omitted. As a rule, conclusions from retrospective studies must be considered to be tentative; they generally can only indicate whether there is any point in pursuing a line of research.

Decide on test instruments needed

To illustrate the difference in response of subjects to Treatment X and Treatment Y, you will have to show the results of some kind of test of their performance. You might have to test your subjects after they receive Treatment X and then after they receive Treatment Y. But the results of receiving Treatment X and then Y would probably be different from receiving only Treatment X or only Treatment Y. Too, the order in which X and Y are received may affect subjects' response. If you gave both tests to all your subjects, you would never know if Treatment X really made all the difference or if you only found better results when you followed it up with Treatment Y. There are many ways, some simple, some extremely complicated, to handle the problem of one treatment influencing the next (see chapter 7). A simple solution is to use two groups of subjects. Give one group Treatment X and the other Treatment Y.

This solves the problem only if the groups were alike in the first place. If they were not, the success of Treatment X may be mostly related to the type of subjects in its group. Worse still, if the subjects were very different from each other, your results might be so garbled that it would be impossible to find any differences at all between the results with one treatment and the results with the other.

This brings up one of the most important concepts in research with human beings: the need to control some variables. *Control* means providing a standard against which to compare the effect of a particular variable (McBurney, 1983). You cannot control all variables, but you can go a long way toward controlling the important ones and eliminating the extraneous ones. Your use of testing instruments will help you do this.

You can control the variables of age and sex either by limiting your groups to one sex and a specified age range – for example, men between the ages of 18 and 23 – or by having "matched groups": For each 19-year-old man in one group, there is a 19-year-old man in the other group.

You may have other criteria for selecting your subjects, such as diagnosis, intelligence level, a specified educational level, marital status, health record, or a specific psychiatric history like a record of previous hospitalization. In the serum chemical studies, we found that college class, age, grades, major course of study, and other variables were correlated with serum chemical levels. It was useful to look at these factors as well as at the football players' positions on the team in studying their serum chemical responses to the football season. Wherever there is an established psychological, biochemical, physical, or other test that will suit your purposes, by all means use that test. Scores of tests standardized on thousands of subjects will make your results more reliable and your work easier to interpret. For other variables, such as demographic, economic, marital, and sociological factors, a simple question-and-answer sheet will serve the purpose, since these variables are well defined and discrete – a woman either is or is not a primipara – and it is easy enough to include or eliminate her on the basis of a simple yes or no response. Make up a form listing all such variables that will allow you to select the appropriate type of subjects, and name the form so you can later refer to it when writing up your research. Then use and preserve the form in obtaining and listing such information on everyone included and excluded from the study. This then becomes one of your *test instruments.*

So far, you have used test instruments only to determine who will be in the samples selected for your study. Now you need a test to determine whether or not Treatment X is really different from Treatment Y. More on this subject will appear in later chapters.

Design the study

Once you have decided on the type of subjects and test instruments you will use, you need to determine how many groups to use and who will administer the tests and treatments. You need to decide before you begin your study whether to control for the effects of time or whether you will be using it as a variable.

Your purposes in setting up the exact design of the research are as follows:

1. To match your experimental and control research groups as well as possible.

2. To make certain that the same procedures are administered to all subjects in your research except the experimental procedure which you administer to a previously specified group or groups.

3. To eliminate as many extraneous variables as possible. In many studies you first need to obtain a *baseline* against which to compare the change in behavior resulting from your drug, behavioral, or other treatment. You measure the patient first for a predetermined period of time in an untreated state – Condition A. This gives you a reference point for assessing the effectiveness of your treatment. Then you administer the drug or other treatment for the same period of time – Condition B. After measuring the effects of your treatment you should, whenever possible, assess your patients again after withdrawing the treatment; that is, return to Condition A. If the behavior then returns toward the baseline, the inference is strengthened that your treatment and not some other variables produced the change. This process is called an *ABA design.* If you then restore the treatment you produce an *ABAB design.* For example, repeated measures of the spring and fall serum uric acid and cholesterol levels of football players produce an increasingly strong test of the research hypothesis. ABA and ABAB designs are often used in single-patient researches.

There are some ethical problems with ABA and ABAB designs with psychiatric patients. First, you may not wish to delay treatment and obtain a pretreatment baseline, Condition A, with desperately ill suicidal or anorexic patients. Likewise, you may wish to continue treatment and not withdraw it from patients undergoing very serious or potentially fatal illnesses that would intensify if you stopped treatment and returned them to pretreatment Condition A. You can sometimes resolve the latter dilemma by cutting back moderately in the treatment and observing the patient's behavior begin to return toward the baseline. Then you can restore the full treatment.

4. To standardize research procedures whether they are given by your-self, your colleagues, your assistants, or anyone else. This is to eliminate *experimenter bias*. If research procedures are not standardized, then those who believe strongly in a procedure, such as Treatment X, might inad-vertently make it work better. Likewise, those who believe in Treatment Y may be able – unconsciously – to influence the results of that treatment. Therefore, standardization of treatment procedures sometimes requires a *blind* or *double-blind design* (see chapter 7). The purpose of these designs is to determine that subjects, researchers, and research helpers are unaware of which subjects are receiving which treatments. These tech-niques are often used in drug studies, where they prevent even the chief experimenter from knowing at the time of administering a dosage whether that dosage is the drug being investigated or a placebo.

5. To decide on what measures will be taken. As a result of your research you must come out with some numbers. For example, the mean serum uric acid (SUA) level of the football players whose blood was drawn during spring training was 5.85, whereas when their blood was drawn in the fall football season it was 6.64. These numbers can be treated statistically to show whether or not these differences are *signifi-cant* (see chapter 4). Statistically significant results imply that your research hypothesis was substantially correct, that your work is meaning-ful and important to your profession, and that it is likely to be published. (In the football players' example, the difference between the spring and fall SUA levels was significant.)

Something must be measured in a defined way if you are to obtain con-vincing evidence that you have tested your contention that Group A is truly different from Group B – or any other hypothesis. And it must be possible for you to communicate exactly how these measurements were made so that another researcher may duplicate or enlarge upon your work. The measurements may be laboratory test findings, number of crying spells over a specified period of time, ratings on a standardized scale, or clinical judgments by therapists regarding a patient's emotional state. They must, however, result eventually in numbers that can be transformed later for use in arithmetic operations. Time spent in defining your crucial measurements well, and in making them concrete, will pay off in time saved when you are ready to analyze your research results.

Decide what statistics you will use

The decision about what statistical treatment you will use must be made before the data are collected. Since collecting data is always the expensive and time-consuming part of research, you will want to be sure that your data are usable after you go to the trouble of accumulating them. For example, if you decide to use a questionnaire where you want to find out the changes in affect, one of the questions on it may be "How are you feeling today?" The answers you receive from your patients will take such forms as "Fine," "Depressed," "OK," "Downhearted," "Nervous," "Blue," "Upset," "Jumpy," and so on. Individuals will express themselves in their own manner, and there will be no way to group their answers together to summarize your results.

Instead, it would be better to supply a set of answers where your patients must choose a response from a list of answers ranging from "Excellent" to "Very depressed." Ahead of time, you will have marked off points on this scale and assigned a rank order to them as follows:

Excellent = 1 Very good = 2 Good = 3 All right = 4 Not so good = 5 A little depressed = 6 Very depressed = 7

Notice that this ordering represents a bipolar scale ranging from one extreme to the other, and that there is a "neutral" midpoint at 4. Your information can now be summarized and treated statistically because you have eliminated the use of an open-ended question where the subjects are allowed to write in any answer they choose. Answers to open-ended questions are the bane of research; they often make the resulting data unusable. You may want an even more refined scale than the seven-point one illustrated above on which to record your data (see chapter 4).

Thus, to save yourself time, expense, and frustration, it is necessary to consider the type of measurement you will use – and therefore the statistical treatment – before you start to collect the data. The chapters that follow describe various kinds of statistics and how to use them.

Decide how many patients/subjects you will use

There is no point in using 500 patients when you could make your point
with 30. Remember that you will have selected a sample to represent a
population. Although case studies have value in their own right, they are
too specific to the individual(s) reported on to be generalizable to a large
group of people. (This problem is similar to the one posed above with the
group of Swedish women.) How many patients, then, are enough – not
too few to be generalizable, and not so many as to waste resources of time
and money?

In general, the finer the scale you use for your measurements and the
more alike the patients are, the fewer patients you will need. If you could
use a scale as fine as that used for many physical measurements (e.g.,
height or weight), and if you could also rule out all extraneous pretest
differences between your subjects, you could use the minimum number
of patients required by the most powerful statistics. However, psychiatric
variables usually cannot be measured in the fine terms of physical ones.
Sometimes the best one can do is to put them on a rank-ordered scale as
shown above. This may limit the researcher in this field to a less powerful
statistic and force the use of larger samples.

For studies using continuous variables (measures having the infinitely
divisible property that the measurement of height or weight has), there is
a simple formula to determine the number of subjects necessary for a
specified degree of precision. However, it requires a close estimate of the
variability within each subject group, as well as other parameters, most
of which are not easily obtainable in new research situations.

It is therefore necessary to use rules of thumb. If you are using a continuous measure, and therefore a parametric statistic (see chapter 4), you
should use no fewer than 10 patients in each group to obtain the highest
power of the applicable parametric statistic. (*Power* means the probability
that a statistical test will find a significant difference when there is in fact
a difference in the sample.) If you are using nominal, rank-ordered, or
ordinal scale measures (chapter 4 provides a discussion of these scales),
you can usually get a value of the statistic with a minimum of 10 patients
per group, but you will get better results if you use as many more than
that as your time and other resources will afford, up to about 20 or 25.
There is always the chance that you will lose some subjects during the
course of the experiment for any one of the multitude of reasons characteristic of human beings. So never start your study with just the mini-

mum allowable number. However, there is a diminishing return from increasing the number of subjects. Doubling the number reduces the error of measurement by only 30%.

A look at the table of values for each statistic in the Appendix will show that, for most, the value is different depending on the number of subjects or degrees of freedom (*df,* which will be explained later). Below the lowest number in the table, the statistic does not apply, so you can let this indicator be your guide.

In general, it is usually not safe to have fewer than 10 subjects per group (either the experimental or the control group). Some statistics will make further breakdowns of your original groups so that you may end up with as few as 5 in a certain cell during the computations. When you get below 5 subjects in a cell or 10 subjects in a major group of your research, you may run into difficulty evaluating the results. This is why you should be sure that your total number of subjects is sufficiently large to accommodate those guidelines.

Single-patient research

Clinical researchers occasionally use single patients to demonstrate the effects of a treatment, especially in behavior management studies. When a treatment causes a large effect, you can profit by studying it with one patient. However, you cannot use statistics with a single patient, since statistics apply only to groups. You or others will eventually want to study your findings with a larger sample of patients. When there are only small differences between the treatment and control conditions, you must increase the size of the sample to increase the probability of obtaining a significant result. Use ABA and ABAB designs whenever possible in single-patient research.

Naturalistic observations

These are defined as observational studies of subjects in their natural environment carried out so as not to disturb the subjects (McBurney, 1983). You prospectively plan to assess responses to certain activities, such as college football games, examinations, and other occurrences. You select a sample in advance and measure before-and-after responses of your subjects. However, you do not randomly assign who does or does not play in both the spring and the fall.

Case studies

You may observe an event involving a single patient or a group of persons; for example, an outbreak of faint-headedness or dizziness in a high school class or factory, or the effects of a disaster such as an earthquake. You had not planned in advance to conduct the research, but you recognize that you must immediately take advantage of the opportunity or lose your chance. Since you have no advance knowledge about when a disaster will occur or who will be a victim, you can only analyze differences among the subjects retrospectively. Case studies differ from naturalistic observations in that the latter are prospective studies, whereas case studies must necessarily be retrospective studies. After the event you can administer tests and questionnaires to both the patient(s) and a comparison group of persons in the class or other setting who did not react abnormally. You report on your hypothesis and the differences you found in support of it.

Obtain permission to conduct research with human subjects, if necessary

There is an elaborate procedure for obtaining permission from hospitals' review boards for research on human subjects, and for asking for informed consent from the patients involved. The process is especially important with patients who enter new treatment or testing programs or where there may be potential risks or discomforts (see chapter 9).

However, in some settings research can proceed without consent. When conducting the research with college football players described here, we were working in a college setting. The student football players were required to undergo complete physical examinations and laboratory testing twice a year, at spring practice and at the competitive fall football season. To obtain serum chemical data for analysis involved no special informed-consent procedure other than to keep confidential all identifiers: players' names, social security numbers, and other personal information.

Determine what other resources you will need

It is important to anticipate all your needs before starting the study. Stumbling upon them while it is in progress may cause you to pass up available patients or may even threaten the successful completion of your work. A mental walkthrough of your proposed research is necessary to reveal what other resources you may need, such as the time of ancillary personnel to administer tests, computer time, expert advice on statistical treatment of data, recording devices, equipment, patient records, colleagues' judgments of patients' progress, or anything else beyond your own time and effort. To be sure there are no hidden surprises, it is useful to conduct a pilot study first.

Pilot studies

Occasionally you may plan a major prospective research of a new test or treatment program. You want to try it out with perhaps hundreds of patients and with many professional and paraprofessional colleagues, and must spend a considerable amount of time, money, and energy. You would be wise first to conduct a pilot study.

In a pilot study you pretest or test out your procedures, instruments, and methods on a small sample of patients. In this small preliminary investigation you can find out whether there are problems in carrying out any of the 15 steps in your research. You can then modify the experimental design and work the bugs out of the procedures before going ahead with the full-scale study. You may also find out from the pilot study whether your hypothesis has any merit and whether the study is worth further time and expense.

Make up data-collection forms

Whether you are planning to conduct a survey, structured interview, systematic behavioral observation, or physiological or chemical analysis, you will need to develop your data-collection form. It must accomplish three purposes. It must provide you and others working with you with (1) an accurate, easy-to-use instrument for recording data; (2) a form that is easy to read, understand, and follow; and (3) reliable and valid information about the matter which you are studying.

First, you need to identify each patient or experimental subject. Researchers often use as a means of quickly spotting a card the first four letters of the subjects' last names along with their first initial. They use a six-digit hospital record or other unique number as their main identifier.

Important demographic information comes next. The data you need vary with the nature of your research. Decide in advance what is important and give yourself the correct number of spaces on your form. Include age (two spaces), sex (one space), and race (three or more spaces). Now provide space for entering the data on the variables you plan to collect.

You may at this point need to train some helpers to do some of the interviewing or testing for you. If so, make certain that they all use the standardized forms and methods you have set up and prepared so that the data collected will be uniform and unbiased.

Collect data

Your research design has been carefully laid out like a set of engineering plans for building a house; you may have conducted a pilot study; and you are now ready to execute your full-scale research. If this is the case, the rest of the work will be interesting, gratifying, and for the most part easy.

Do arithmetic analyses

You will be able to perform most statistical analyses of the kind discussed here with a hand calculator and the formulas discussed in chapters 4.A and 5.A. However, if you have a great many data, or the statistic requires a number of mathematical steps, you will want to do your work or have it done on a computer, since this process is faster, more accurate, and less expensive than any hand calculations.

If the statistical test has been applied and you find that it has rejected the null hypothesis, this means that your research hypothesis has a high probability of being correct. You now have a credible research finding, and you are ready to write it up for presentation at a professional gathering, submit it to a professional journal, or both.

But what do you do if the statistical test does not reject the null hypothesis? Or, put another way, if the statistical test in effect states that it found no difference between two treatments – or any other two variables that you thought were different? There are a number of possibilities for making good use of the work you have done:

1. Sometimes it is important to know that the effects of two different variables are the same. Consider, for example, the use of two different drugs. Suppose one is expensive and the other is not. If there is no difference in the results they produce, then there is every reason to prefer the less expensive one. This is important information.

Or if two popular treatments exist to alleviate the same symptom where one treatment requires three years to be effective and the other takes only six months, again the information is useful.

2. You may have used too few patients to show a treatment difference. The effect you are after may be so subtle that it is obscured by the individual differences among subjects that you could not control. If this is true, it may show up more clearly if you add more patients to the study. Adding more patients may (depending on what measures you are using; see chapter 4) enable you to use a more powerful statistic, that is, one that will detect more subtle differences.

3. Your research may contradict a similar one already in the literature. Your original literature search will already have told you that someone else had an idea similar to yours and did find a difference between the treatment variables. If you performed an exact duplicate of that person's research and found no difference, then this is important information to your colleagues – given that your research was conducted under rigorous scientific conditions. If, on the other hand, your research purposely incorporated (or left out) some of the variables used by the previous researcher, then this information is extremely valuable. It indicates that the treatment is effective under certain conditions but ineffective under the conditions you employed.

4. Your research hypothesis is wrong. This is always a possibility. However, such hypotheses, or educated guesses, usually have a germ of validity. If you have been in practice over a period of years and have noticed a certain tendency in your patients, it is very likely that there is something there. Your research design, or your statistic, may not have been powerful enough to measure it, but that may not mean that it does not exist. In this case, it is often helpful to discuss your entire project with a knowledgeable colleague or with an expert in experimental design and statistics. All universities and many colleges include several such experts on their faculties. You will very likely find that one of these professionals is willing to review your work and determine whether or not useful information can be teased out of it. Sometimes a consulting fee will be requested; other times the consultant will ask only to be included as a coauthor of your research report. If you have put a great deal of time and effort into the work and still feel that in some way your hunch is correct, it is certainly worth submitting to such an expert for review.

Write up results

Given that your work produced results that have some scientific value (either by confirming or rejecting your research hypothesis), you are now in the enjoyable position of being ready to write up the results. The microcomputer can help you here as a word processor. When you have data to report, you will need to use tables and graphs. A few words on this subject follow.

Using tables

Tables present data that describe important details about your subjects or patients and what happened to them in your study. Since readers will pay special attention to them, make sure they express clearly what you are presenting. They should include (1) the number of subjects, (2) the tests performed, (3) the before-and-after conditions of the study and their numerical data, (4) the statistical tests and their results, and (5) the probabilities of occurrence by chance.

Format of a research paper

There is a standardized format for reporting results of quantitative measurement, observed relation, and causal relation research. Ideally, a research paper uses minimal space to report maximal necessary information. Each report contains a title, an initial abstract, an introduction, a statement of the problem, a methods section, a results section, a discussion, and a bibliography. Some journals require a summary, but one may not be necessary when a good abstract is available.

The *title* is an important part of every paper, chapter, or book. It is the first thing that readers see; it can stir their interest or turn them off. Here are some questions to ask yourself about the title you give your paper. Is it short enough? Does it tell what your report is about? Does it catch potential readers' attention?

The *abstract* should tell clearly and simply what you did and what you found in under 100 words (40–50 words in the case of brief clinical or research reports). Most readers look at the abstract before they read the article. If they are confused by what they see, you have lost them before they even begin to read your article.

The *introduction* need not be given a heading. It should be as brief as possible.

State the problem concisely so that your readers have a frame of reference for comprehending what follows. Review thoroughly what has been published (by yourself and others) in the specific area of investigation. Provide information on classic and current writings on the subject, and clarify what is accepted as valid and where there are weaknesses.

Present your research hypothesis clearly and your reasons for attacking it. Many of the points made earlier about initial working hypotheses apply here.

Failure to refer to important research in the field may have dire consequences. Persons who are asked to review submitted articles know a good deal about the subject on which you have written. Frequently they have published papers in the field. If you do not discuss some important reports in the literature, journal editors and reviewers may develop a bias against your study that may prevent them from accepting it.

The *methods and procedures* section provides a detailed explanation of your research design, including the following:

1. Number and type of subjects, controls, or comparison groups
2. Instruments used (screening tests, interviews, etc.)
3. Treatments and other procedures used (experimental tests, drugs, therapies, etc.)
4. Variables studied (independent, dependent, intervening, extraneous, controlled, or uncontrolled)
5. Methods of collecting data
6. Statistical tests used

The *results* section tells what happened when your statistics were applied to the data you gathered. Work hard at making your tables and graphs clearly understandable and attractive. Experienced readers study the results section carefully. You may also wish to present some qualitative information here – pictures, case histories, excerpts from tape recordings. Think of the *Scientific American*. Do you frequently go through its articles looking not only at the tables and graphs but also at the pictures? Good qualitative pictures of brain images or patients' appearance, posture, and expression, for example, can complement quantitative data. Qualitative material such as verbal content of interviews, facial expression at different periods of treatment, or anatomical structures in the brain may also, like X rays, be subjected to quantitative measurement and analysis.

The *discussion and conclusions* section gives you freedom to consider the implications of your findings. Here you can speculate as to causality. If there are other reports that your findings confirm or do not confirm, this is the place to say so. If you discovered during the course of your work that some other variables, which your study was not set up to investigate, might be relevant, point this out here. If there is a controversy in the literature about some aspect of the topic you are addressing, then show what light your work sheds on that controversy. Include here what form you feel follow-up studies should take in the future. If you think other similar studies erred in some way, you may state your opinion here. In short, the report of your work must be objective in every other section of the article, but your own opinions are appropriate in the discussion. State your conclusions in consideration of all you have said in the discussion.

Last, whereas literary quality is usually not an important consideration in the evaluation of a submitted journal article, clarity is. Many more articles are submitted than are printed. Brevity is therefore always desirable, and a clear, concise description of your work is essential.

The *summary* briefly restates your research hypothesis and summarizes the results of your work.

The *bibliography* lists all references to the published work of others as well as to any previous work of your own on this topic. (Journals differ widely in the form used for citing references. To avoid time-consuming rewriting, follow their printed directions closely.) You may also refer to unpublished work when necessary.

Be prepared for the fact that it may take some time for the journal of your choice to evaluate your article and advise you whether or not it intends to accept it. Most reputable publications send submitted articles to at least one and as many as three experts in the area of your research. All of these must fit their review of your work into their daily schedules. It may take several months for these expert opinions to arrive back at the editor's desk and for him to make a decision based on them. After an article is accepted by a journal, it may still take anywhere from six months to two years for it to appear in print.

Oral reports

Since it may take more than a year for a paper to be published, you will reach your audience much sooner by presenting your research findings at one of the numerous psychiatric meetings held each year. Oral reports contain the same sections as written papers. But there are differences:

1. Make your oral report short, since you will have only 10 to 15 minutes in which to make your presentation.

2. Make it simple, so that your listeners can understand it while you are talking.

3. Do not bore your readers by reading your report; deliver it from an outline.

4. Make only one or two points in each of the sections.

5. Make the introduction, methods, and discussion sections especially brief.

6. Emphasize the results. They are what interest your listeners the most.

7. Use visual aids – slides or overhead transparencies. Make the printing large and legible. Avoid complicated tables.

8. Summarize your findings at the end of your presentation.

Summary

This chapter has completed a discussion of the steps needed for setting up, executing, and publishing the results of a research study. Where further detail is needed, it has referred you to later chapters of this book. The chapter explained the format of written and oral research reports.

4. Research to develop measuring instruments

To determine the degree of validity of a concept, you must be able to measure it reliably. Research to develop measuring instruments (or measurement research) is concerned with whether and how well a test or instrument measures a concept. By *measurement* we mean the process of assigning numbers to objects or events according to rules (McBurney, 1983).

Definition

A concept has reached the measurement research stage if it has fulfilled the following criteria:

1. It can be defined operationally
2. There is a specifiable technique for measuring it
3. There is agreement on the outcomes of measurement

The concept has won acceptance because it has been shown to be reliable. In clinical settings, measurement research is concerned with the clinical applicabiity of the concept and its tests.

Using clinical tests

In performing a clinical test you take measurements in a systematic, consistent manner, holding conditions as constant as possible. All systematic observations – taking a patient's history, conducting a laboratory assay, performing a physical or mental examination – are kinds of clinical tests. The usefulness of new clinical tests is investigated by measurement research. This chapter describes measurement research and shows how to quantify information that you collect from patients and how to begin to analyze it statistically.

Measurement research follows the 15 steps discussed previously. The present and subsequent chapters do not repeat details of research steps presented in earlier sections, but only go through and explain the new procedures needed.

Some of the measurement research presented here examines the usefulness and clinical applicability of two concepts and their measures: aggravating stress (measured by the Axis IV scale of the third edition of the American Psychiatric Association's *Diagnostic and Statistical Manual of Mental Disorders – DSM-III* [1980]) and premorbid functioning level (*DSM-III*'s Axis V scale). The reliability of these two *DSM-III* quantitative scales was tested and reported in *DSM-III*. Our studies looked at their usefulness and validity. They explored relationships between scores on these measures and inpatients' length of hospital stay, testing the research hypothesis that Axis IV and Axis V are related to the amount of treatment that psychiatric inpatients need.

This chapter also describes the process of developing a new questionnaire or survey form. To develop a new measuring instrument – whether it be biochemical, physical, physiological, or psychosocial – involves a number of steps: measuring validity, reliability, selectivity, and sensitivity; and, with psychosocial tests and questionnaires, selecting and analyzing test items. Let us now define and discuss some of these terms as they apply to psychiatric tests and instruments.

More definitions

Objectivity is the use of methods that eliminate the subjective by limiting choices to fixed alternatives requiring a minimum of creative interpretation.

Standardization is the process of making all similar data-gathering or test instruments the same so that all data or test results for a designated research project are obtained in exactly the same way no matter how many different persons collect the information.

Validity is the fidelity with which a clinical test assesses whatever it purports to assess. Validity implies support by objective evidence. There are three major kinds of validity: content validity, criterion-related validity, and construct validity. To establish content validity of a test, you demonstrate that all its items measure the same subject matter. To measure criterion-related validity, you show that scores on the test correlate with independent measures of the same concept. Frequently findings from a new instrument are compared with those from an established one to determine the former's criterion-related validity. To demonstrate construct validity, you show that in controlled studies the test measures what you might hypothesize it to do. For example, the *DSM-III* quantitative studies above examined the hypothesis that chronic long-term inpatients' Axis V scores are worse than those of short-term inpatients and the latter's scores are worse than those of outpatients. Thus this research tested the construct validity of the Axis V premorbid functional level scale.

A cross-validation occurs when the validity of a new clinical test obtained in a first study is checked in a second and later studies. The data in Tables 4.2 and 4.3 came from a cross-validation (Larsen et al., 1966) – a replication of earlier measurement research using the same instrument, the maternity questionnaire, with different subjects in another setting.

Reliability is the ability of a clinical test consistently to measure the same objects or events as long as it is being administered, from beginning to end, and to yield the same results on repeated tests by the same researcher or others. You obtain test–retest reliability by repeating a test and measuring the correlation between the two results. Some tests have two or more parallel, equivalent, or alternate forms. By using different forms with a patient, you avoid the possible practice effect that occurs when you repeat the same test. You measure the test–retest reliability of the hospital's equipment by correlating the results with different forms with each other.

As part of their quality assurance procedure, hospitals call upon outside testing agencies to recalibrate their X ray and ECG equipment periodically, and to retest blood and other samples from their clinical laboratories at regular intervals in order to determine the reliability of their own measurements. Likewise, clinicians periodically repeat blood pressure readings or pulse rate counts to test the reliability of their own or their assistants' measurements. Interjudge reliability measures how closely two judges or two groups of judges agree in their judgments, ratings, or other decisions.

The unreliability of patients' memories of events in their personal health histories is well known. That is why you routinely request reports from other physicians and hospitals about patients' tests, medications, and illnesses, and speak to other members of their families, rather than rely entirely upon patients' personal statements. When you look at the reports, you do not as a rule calculate a correlation, but you nevertheless determine in your mind how reliable are patients' statements about dates of treatments and other data. Many psychiatrists and other physicians protect themselves from expensive and painful malpractice suits by checking patients' reports. By performing your own examinations of the patient, you can gauge the reliability of historical reports; by checking with the pharmacist, you learn how reliable your patients' statements about specific medications are.

Researchers measure the reliability of psychiatric tests and instruments by repeating the use of the same instrument and determining the correspondence between the readings. With psychosocial instruments, this procedure may sometimes be feasible in a research setting, but sometimes problems arise when patients must retake a psychological test or instrument. Then researchers use alternate or parallel forms of a psychological test.

Norms are how a large number of people perform on a test under standard conditions. Norms let you know what a particular score means and what to expect when you use the test in the future.

Getting subjects for research

A good place to find research subjects is in any setting where people come together in groups – in your office, the hospitals and clinics with which you are affiliated, the colleges where you consult, and so on.

The research into the usefulness and validity of *DSM-III*'s Axes IV and V used the charts of patients who had been treated in a university hospital's psychiatric outpatient clinic and inpatient unit.

The studies of maternal stresses used psychiatric maternity patients treated in office practice. Normal obstetrical patients who delivered at a local community hospital and psychiatric maternity patients who had been hospitalized in a psychiatric facility served as comparison groups. The psychiatrically hospitalized group was considered to be sicker than those treated as office outpatients. The obstetrical ward group was assumed to be less emotionally ill than the office patients. These studies followed up on the earlier initial working hypothesis research discussed previously.

The term *comparison group*, rather than *control group*, appears in the previous paragraph, because we did not exert control over who entered the maternity ward or psychiatric hospital. When you use a comparison group you must try to match it as well as possible with your experimental group. On the other hand, when you perform a controlled experiment, you actually determine in advance, preselect, and assign persons to be your controls.

Random selection

Random selection is selection conducted in such a way that each member of the population has an equal chance of becoming a member of the sample. In common parlance this term is often used to mean "careless" or "unorganized" or "unplanned" selection, but in statistics it has a precise meaning.

In actual practice, it is not possible to select subjects exactly in accordance with the definition. Very often research is conducted by choosing the first subjects who come along who fit the general description of what you are looking for, are easily available, and are willing to be subjects. For the most part, this works out all right as far as the statistics are concerned. But some selection methods should definitely be avoided. Since it is easier to explain what you should not do under the rubric of random selection than to state practical general rules for what you should do, we shall list the forbidden practices here.

1. You should not select subjects by choosing people who will prove the point you want to make and excluding those who might not. If you do this, then the results of your study apply only to the type of subject you selected, not to the general population you may be interested in.

For example, in some work on preventing the highly stressful crime of rape, one objective was to determine, if possible, what methods (such as screaming, fighting back, pleading, or verbalized defiance) were most effective in preventing a threatened rape attack. Suppose we had decided that the best source of answers to this question would be those women who had been faced with a rapist, yet managed to escape from the situation untouched. It would seem reasonable to assume that we could get the answer from them by finding out what type of resistance they used. This done, suppose we found that the majority of these resisters had physically fought off the rapist. Then we could conclude that a woman's best approach when faced with a rapist would be to fight back physically, and we would publish this advice to all women. But this would be a very dangerous and erroneous conclusion. Why? Because if we had also interviewed the rape victims (or read the police reports about them) we should have found that many of them had also physically grappled with their attackers. Some lost their lives, and all got raped. A closer look at the data for all the subjects, victims and resisters, might show that on the average, the resisters were 50 pounds heavier and five inches taller than the victims. Or that most resisters were accosted by a man who had no weapon, whereas the victims faced an attacker wielding a knife or a gun. Thus, choosing to study only the "good subjects," that is, the rape resisters, would have resulted in our promulgating some tragically false advice. But the fallacy only becomes obvious when all the facts are presented. Many psychiatric variables will be even more deeply hidden and yet just as entangled with the one you want to study.

Keep in mind that some other researcher may do a similar study, using randomly selected subjects, and get a completely different result. This stacking of the deck (consciously or not) can not only ruin your reputation as a researcher but may also have far-reaching or tragic results for the general public.

Since the objective of the study was to establish the facts about rape, it was necessary to use a standardized form to record facts objectively. In this way, preconceived notions about who gets raped or why or when or where were not allowed to enter into the selection of subjects for the study. Had we first taken a viewpoint and then chosen subjects (i.e., rape victims) to fit it, the conclusions emerging from the study (which have been widely used since then to influence legislation across the country) would have promptly been shown to be wrong either by an unbiased researcher or by someone with an opposing viewpoint.

2. Do not use a special group of people as your research sample for reasons of convenience unless you restrict the applicability of your results to a population of such people. For example, in our studies of the EEG of normal sleep, it might have been easier on the technical staff if we had selected only subjects who were willing to do their sleeping in the daytime rather than overnight. But if we had done so, we should then have been able to generalize the results only to daytime sleepers, not to the general population of people who sleep at night. In like manner, since all the studies in the cited population – and many related ones (Hursch, 1970; Hursch, Karacan & Williams, 1972; R. L. Williams, Hursch & Karacan, 1972; R. L. Williams, Karacan & Hursch, 1974) – were for the sake of convenience performed on white subjects, the results may not apply to black persons or to those of any other untested race.

3. Do not fail to set up criteria ahead of time for including subjects in the study (such as age and marital status) and then take every available subject, up to the limit of your sample size, who fits those criteria, regardless of your biases about whether or not that person will or will not be a "good subject." If you prejudge your subjects, you will be introducing bias of some kind whether or not you are aware of it. This may or may not favor your research hypothesis; either way, you run the chance of producing results that may someday embarrass you.

Deciding on clinical test instruments

As discussed before, a physical, biochemical, psychosocial, or other clinical test is standardized when (1) the conditions are defined under which measures are taken and (2) the methods are specified by which scores are derived and interpreted. You can readily compare results with standardized tests. Therefore, use standardized tests, interviews, and instruments developed by others whenever possible, rather than try to design your own. The task of creating a new psychosocial instrument can be time-consuming and tedious, as is shown later.

Some well-known psychiatric instruments for assessing behavior and personality were developed in the 1950s and 1960s for determining the effects of new psychotropic medications. The following are some widely used standardized psychiatric tests and rating scales.

For psychiatric outpatients: the Brief Psychiatric Rating Scale (BPRS) (Overall & Gorham, 1962), the Wittenborn Psychiatric Rating Scale (WPRS) (Wittenborn, 1950), the Hamilton Depression Scale (Hamilton, 1960), the Hamilton Anxiety Scale (Hamilton, 1959), the Diagnostic Interview Schedule (Robins, Helzer, Croughan & Ratcliff, 1981), and the well-known Minnesota Multiphasic Personality Inventory (MMPI) (Greene, 1980).

For psychiatric inpatients: the Inpatient Multidimensional Psychiatric Scale (IMPS) (Lorr, 1953), the Nurses' Observational Scale for Inpatient Evaluation (NOSIE-30) (Honigfeld, Gillis & Klett, 1966), the Discharge Readiness Inventory (DRI) (Hogarty & Ulrich, 1972), and the Structured Clinical Interview (SCI) (Burdock & Hardesty, 1969).

For self-report: the Katz Adjustment Scales (KAS) (Katz & Lyerly, 1963), the Beck Depression Inventory (BDI) (Beck, 1972), and the State–Trait Anxiety Inventory (STAI) (Spielberger, 1968).

Benefits of standardized psychiatric tests and rating scales

The tests above and many other standardized psychiatric tests and rating scales provide you with information about your patients that has been standardized on many other patients and therefore is objective and can be scored easily. The validity and reliability of the scales have already been checked, making it unnecessary for you to repeat the work. Some of these measures, as well as others, have been adapted for use with children. They offer you an opportunity to find out where your own patients stand, either individually or in groups, in comparison either with predetermined norms or with other psychiatric patients. Many are available for microcomputer administration and scoring. Each year computer software for both old and new tests comes on the market. Check the exhibit booths at national psychiatric meetings for the latest offerings.

As research tools, standardized tests will be invaluable to you, since they will serve to establish, for example, base rates of behavior. If you then institute treatments that you think may be effective, it will be possible to show meaningful changes over these base rates if your treatment fulfills the promise you believe it to have. They will also show that your control group was behaviorally the same as your experimental group before you imposed the treatment. In other words, a standardized body of tests such as these eliminates the need for you to engage in the time-consuming and expensive work necessary to set the stage for your research.

With these instruments, you also can assess your individual patient, if you wish, even if you are not conducting a formal research. You can measure a patient's progress or that of groups of patients in a treatment program. You can compare your findings with those you obtained previously or with those of other colleagues and facilities who use the same rating scales. The data you will obtain provide 30 or more different kinds of advantages to patients, therapeutic programs, treatment facilities, and communities, as well as to research, training, and education, as is shown in Table 4.1.

As can be seen in the table, standardized psychiatric rating scales as a group can perform many useful functions in the practice of clinical psychiatry as well as in psychiatric research. However, none alone can do all of the above. For this reason we have sought to develop a comprehensive psychiatric patient rating procedure for both research and clinical purposes to accomplish everything in Table 4.1 (see chapter 8).

Collecting data

If you interview or test groups of patients or other subjects where they naturally gather, such as in your or your colleague's office or in a class, clinic, or hospital, you will save time and money. In the last two cases you may find that the subjects have time on their hands and are eager to cooperate just to keep busy. For example, women on obstetrical wards

Table 4.1. *Advantages of standardized psychiatric tests and rating scales*

A. Patient benefits
 1. Obtaining a standardized, objective record of patient symptoms, behavior, and interview data
 2. Providing easy and accurate scoring
 3. Providing reliable and valid information
 4. Generating computer-assisted information directly from patients
 5. Providing a nonthreatening, inoffensive method of obtaining data
 6. Gaining patients' interest
 7. Obtaining objective information from patients' relatives
 8. Facilitating the interview process
 9. Printing out reports automatically
10. Assessing patients' symptoms – depression, two kinds of anxiety, etc.
11. Helping make a diagnosis
12. Offering presession self-reports to facilitate the therapeutic interview
13. Assessing patient progress in treatment
14. Comparing changes in data from interview to interview
15. Charting progress
16. Providing data and graphs for patients' charts and records
17. Helping plan for discharge
18. Comparing patients' responses with those of norms
19. Measuring patients' prehospital and posthospital adjustment in the community

B. Program and facility benefits
1. Obtaining both patient and normative data
2. Assessing patient progress in programs and facilities
3. Assessing program efficiency
4. Comparing data from one program to another and between facilities

C. Community epidemiological benefits
1. Obtaining both patient and normative data for community epidemiological and other purposes
2. Comparing patients' responses with those of norms
3. Assessing change in communities
4. Providing comparative data for epidemiological study (social indicators) – stress, pathology in the community

D. Research benefits
1. Selecting patients for study
2. Measuring changes in symptoms or behavior of research patients

E. Training and education
1. Helping staff and professionals develop and improve interviewing skills
2. Assessing staff and professional interviewing skills

were very cooperative in filling in a lengthy version of the maternity questionnaire discussed below.

The *DSM-III* Axis IV and Axis V studies used hospital and clinic charts of discharged psychiatric patients whose *DSM-III* scales had previously been rated. This retrospective study cost nothing but time to count numbers and analyze the data by computer.

Data-collection forms

Before beginning your research, make up forms for collecting the data systematically. A computer-generated form for collecting Axis IV and Axis V data from discharged psychiatric inpatients' records appears in Figure 4.1. Note that there is room for data on 50 patients on this form. Other forms such as tally sheets can collect data on thousands of patients on one page. At the other extreme, the maternity questionnaire described later in this chapter, which obtained the information shown below in Tables 4.2 and 4.3, requires many pages for just one patient to fill in her personal history.

In Figure 4.1 the abbreviation "FL (8 − Axis V)" means premorbid functional level, calculated by transforming the Axis V score by subtracting it from the number 8; "SR (Axis IV/FL)" means the strain ratio (which is the ratio of Axis IV to the transformed Axis V score); "Adm" and "Dsch" are the admission and discharge dates; "AMA" means discharged against medical advice; "Othr" means transfer to another hospital; and "LOS (Dsch–Adm)" is the length of hospital stay, calculated by computing the number of days between the day of discharge and the day of admission.

The role of statistics

In doing measurement research, you will be collecting a new type of data resulting from the responses of your research subjects on the specific clinical test you are studying. You will then compare these data with the test responses of a comparison group of subjects or with the research subjects' responses on another validated test or instrument.

You will need to summarize the results. You cannot simply recite all sorts of scores for one group and then for another. This is where statistics comes to the rescue by offering the means to condense and summarize great quantities of data in a few simple descriptive terms. But summarizing is only one of the uses of statistics. Suppose you are able to state that

	Name	Number	Sex	Age	Race	Axis I	Axis II	Axis III	Axis IV	Axis V	FL'(8–Axis V'	SR (Axis IV/FL)	Adm	Dsch	AMA	Othr	LOS (Dsch-Adm)
1	•	•	•	•	•	•	•	•	•	•	•	•	•	•	•	•	•
2	•	•	•	•	•	•	•	•	•	•	•	•	•	•	•	•	•
3	•	•	•	•	•	•	•	•	•	•	•	•	•	•	•	•	•
4	•	•	•	•	•	•	•	•	•	•	•	•	•	•	•	•	•
5	•	•	•	•	•	•	•	•	•	•	•	•	•	•	•	•	•
6	•	•	•	•	•	•	•	•	•	•	•	•	•	•	•	•	•
7	•	•	•	•	•	•	•	•	•	•	•	•	•	•	•	•	•
8	•	•	•	•	•	•	•	•	•	•	•	•	•	•	•	•	•
9	•	•	•	•	•	•	•	•	•	•	•	•	•	•	•	•	•
10	•	•	•	•	•	•	•	•	•	•	•	•	•	•	•	•	•
11	•	•	•	•	•	•	•	•	•	•	•	•	•	•	•	•	•
12	•	•	•	•	•	•	•	•	•	•	•	•	•	•	•	•	•
13	•	•	•	•	•	•	•	•	•	•	•	•	•	•	•	•	•
14	•	•	•	•	•	•	•	•	•	•	•	•	•	•	•	•	•
15	•	•	•	•	•	•	•	•	•	•	•	•	•	•	•	•	•
16	•	•	•	•	•	•	•	•	•	•	•	•	•	•	•	•	•
17	•	•	•	•	•	•	•	•	•	•	•	•	•	•	•	•	•
18	•	•	•	•	•	•	•	•	•	•	•	•	•	•	•	•	•
19	•	•	•	•	•	•	•	•	•	•	•	•	•	•	•	•	•
20	•	•	•	•	•	•	•	•	•	•	•	•	•	•	•	•	•
21	•	•	•	•	•	•	•	•	•	•	•	•	•	•	•	•	•
22	•	•	•	•	•	•	•	•	•	•	•	•	•	•	•	•	•
23	•	•	•	•	•	•	•	•	•	•	•	•	•	•	•	•	•
24	•	•	•	•	•	•	•	•	•	•	•	•	•	•	•	•	•
25	•	•	•	•	•	•	•	•	•	•	•	•	•	•	•	•	•
26	•	•	•	•	•	•	•	•	•	•	•	•	•	•	•	•	•
27	•	•	•	•	•	•	•	•	•	•	•	•	•	•	•	•	•
28	•	•	•	•	•	•	•	•	•	•	•	•	•	•	•	•	•
29	•	•	•	•	•	•	•	•	•	•	•	•	•	•	•	•	•
30	•	•	•	•	•	•	•	•	•	•	•	•	•	•	•	•	•
31	•	•	•	•	•	•	•	•	•	•	•	•	•	•	•	•	•
32	•	•	•	•	•	•	•	•	•	•	•	•	•	•	•	•	•
33	•	•	•	•	•	•	•	•	•	•	•	•	•	•	•	•	•
34	•	•	•	•	•	•	•	•	•	•	•	•	•	•	•	•	•
35	•	•	•	•	•	•	•	•	•	•	•	•	•	•	•	•	•
36	•	•	•	•	•	•	•	•	•	•	•	•	•	•	•	•	•
37	•	•	•	•	•	•	•	•	•	•	•	•	•	•	•	•	•
38	•	•	•	•	•	•	•	•	•	•	•	•	•	•	•	•	•
39	•	•	•	•	•	•	•	•	•	•	•	•	•	•	•	•	•
40	•	•	•	•	•	•	•	•	•	•	•	•	•	•	•	•	•
41	•	•	•	•	•	•	•	•	•	•	•	•	•	•	•	•	•
42	•	•	•	•	•	•	•	•	•	•	•	•	•	•	•	•	•
43	•	•	•	•	•	•	•	•	•	•	•	•	•	•	•	•	•
44	•	•	•	•	•	•	•	•	•	•	•	•	•	•	•	•	•
45	•	•	•	•	•	•	•	•	•	•	•	•	•	•	•	•	•
46	•	•	•	•	•	•	•	•	•	•	•	•	•	•	•	•	•
47	•	•	•	•	•	•	•	•	•	•	•	•	•	•	•	•	•
48	•	•	•	•	•	•	•	•	•	•	•	•	•	•	•	•	•
49	•	•	•	•	•	•	•	•	•	•	•	•	•	•	•	•	•
50	•	•	•	•	•	•	•	•	•	•	•	•	•	•	•	•	•

Figure 4.1. Microcomputer-generated form for collecting Axis IV and Axis V scores. Each sheet will contain the title of the research (e.g., "*DSM-III* Axes IV and V Research"), the date, the recorder of data, the patient group, and a page number.

the average score of one group is greater than, or less than, the average score of the other group. You are still in the dark about whether or not the difference is meaningful. After all, the unusual finding would probably be that both means are exactly the same! Therefore, how much different do they have to be for the difference to have occurred for some reason other than chance? You would have no meaningful way to answer this question if it were not for the development of the science of statistical inference.

Fortunately, in recent years many statistics have been invented specifically for use with psychosocial variables, which are often not as concrete as variables in some of the physical sciences. These statistics serve both descriptive and inferential purposes. Many are so easy to compute that you can do it yourself with pencil, paper, and a hand calculator. We show you how to use them here and present examples of clinical research that applied them. Software programs for most others are now available for your home or office microcomputer. However, statistical complexity ranges all the way from the simple ones above to some that require a large computer, so it is well to understand the statistic you will use before you start.

Chapters 4.A and 5.A show the computation of most of the statistics you will need in studying your own patients and in conducting special studies such as those described in this book. They also list the conditions necessary for the use of each statistic. Unless you have an urge to know more about the derivation or the mathematical assumptions underlying a statistic, there is no need to go into these topics. (We refer anyone interested to the references mentioned in chapter 5.A under "Suggestions for Further Reading.") It is usually sufficient to know the conditions under which a statistic may be used and how to compute it. However, three general properties of numbers should be kept in mind by anyone approaching a research study. These are (1) types of variables, (2) types of measurement scales, and (3) types of statistics. A brief discussion of these topics follows.

Types of variables

All variables occur in one or the other of the following two forms:

1. A *discrete variable,* such as number of hospital admissions, is one that falls into separate categories with no possible intermediate values (McBurney, 1983). This is always a whole number. If we plotted number

of admissions for each member of a group of subjects, we would plot whole numbers such as 9, 2, 0, 4, 8. There is no such thing as half an admission or two-thirds of one. To express this concept more generally, there are no points on our scale between the integers. Contrast this with the next type of variable.

2. A *continuous variable,* such as weight, is one that falls along a continuum and is not limited to a certain number of values (McBurney, 1983). The weight of an adult is usually expressed in a whole number, e.g., 134 lb, but this actually means "over 133.9 lb but under 135 lb." For a neonate, weight may be stated as $7\frac{1}{2}$ lb, which is still not exactly correct but puts the measurement in a smaller interval: "somewhere between 7.25 and 7.75 lb." For a premature infant, weight may be stated in ounces. For a laboratory animal such as a white rat, weight is expressed in grams. And we can go down the scale as far as our measuring instruments will allow, until we are stating weight in numbers of atoms. We could go further down if we had the instruments to measure it. To put this concept in precise terms: The distance between any two points on the scale of weights is infinitely divisible; that is, no matter how finely we divide the interval between the two points, we will achieve another meaningful number by dividing it again. Such a variable is called continuous.

Types of scales

Another important consideration is the type of scale you use for your measurements. All measurements will result in numbers, but these numbers will have different properties. The statistic you use depends on the properties your numbers have. Your numbers will constitute one of the following types of scales:

1. *Nominal.* Here the numbers are only names; they serve only to identify categories of similar or different objects or events. You cannot use arithmetic on them. The numbers on a football player's back are in this category. (Since ends are often given numbers in the 80s and halfbacks in the 40s, do you get two backs by dividing an end by 2?) In psychiatric nomenclature, *DSM-III*'s Axes I, II, and III, but not its Axes IV and V, are all on nominal scales.

If you are plotting the progress of 10 of your patients for comparison later, you may, to obscure their identity, record them as Pt 1, Pt 2, and so on, up to Pt 10. But these numbers are only labels. You may arrange them on a line, but the relationship of each patient to each other patient on that line has no meaning – Pt 3 is not better than nor worse off than Pt 4. However, there is a group of statistics you may use on them, called *nonparametric* statistics, which will be discussed briefly at the end of this section. You can also accumulate frequencies on this nominal scale, and the frequencies are real numbers obeying the rules of arithmetic. The frequencies may be subjected to more high-powered statistics than nonparametrics.

2. *Ordinal.* Ordinal numbers are those whose position on the scale is meaningful, but which do not necessarily have the same amount of space between them. They arrange events or objects in order of their magnitude. For example, if you took the 10 patients mentioned above and ordered them according to the severity of their symptoms, with Pt 1 being the most severely ill and Pt 10 the least severely ill, the numbers would then take on a new meaning: Pt 1 is the sickest, Pt 2 is the second sickest, and so on. Socioeconomic status is also measured on an ordinal scale. An ordinal scale is *rank-ordered,* and though you still cannot apply arithmetic to the numbers, they have acquired a new quality.

Note that the intervals between numbers may not be equal – Pt 3 may be in almost as bad condition as Pt 2 while the difference between the conditions of Pts 4 and 5 may be great. All that is implied as you go up the scale is that the patient with the higher number is better off than the one with the lower number. There are nonparametric statistical tests with which you can handle data arranged on rank-ordered, or ordinal, scales.

3. *Interval.* On this scale, the distances between points are equal. An example of this is a centigrade or a Fahrenheit thermometer. One degree is the same size whether it is the degree from 32 to 33 or the one from 104 to 105. This same assumption underlies tests like I.Q. scales. However, in both of those temperature scales and the I.Q. scale, there is no meaningful zero point. We do not mean "no intelligence" at the zero point on an I.Q. scale, any more than we mean "no temperature" when we reach the zero point on the centigrade or Fahrenheit scale. Interval scales are more precise or refined than ordinal and nominal ones.

With most interval scales, it is possible to use parametric statistics, Pearson correlations, the *t* test, the *F* test, and so on, because the laws of arithmetic do apply. In general, a parametric test should be used wherever possible because of its higher power. But for many types of data, such as those measured on nominal and ordinal scales, there are no parametric statistical tests available. Many physiological and biochemical measures are on interval scales. Psychologists and other social scientists, who construct psychosocial instruments like intelligence tests, usually develop them with interval scales. When you work with a psychosocial test, check whether it has an interval or an ordinal scale, so you will know what kind of statistics to use with it – parametric or nonparametric.

4. *Ratio.* This scale has all the properties of the scales above, as well as a meaningful zero point. For example, the Kelvin scale for measuring temperature, unlike the centigrade and Fahrenheit scales, does have a meaningful zero point (at -273 °C or -458 °F), called absolute zero, and therefore constitutes a ratio scale. You can use the highest-powered parametric statistics on the numbers on this scale, given that your data conform to the other requirements of the statistic you choose.

Types of statistical tests

The *power* of a statistical test is the probability that it will detect a difference between two sets of data when a difference actually exists. The power of a test may be increased to some extent by increasing the number of subjects tested.

1. *Parametric.* This is a group of tests of differences between groups of data that make use of parametric statistics like mean, standard deviation, and variance. Parametric statistics are based on the assumption of defined distribution (usually the normal distribution) for the underlying population. A parametric test will allow you to make a statement about the probability that your two sets of data – one for the treatment group and one for the comparison group – are or are not significantly different. In other words, you will be able to state the probability that the results are due to the treatment you used rather than due to chance. (For convenience, we discuss these points in terms of a comparison between two groups, but the comparison could be between several groups.) Parametric statistical tests include Student's *t* test, the *F* test for analysis of variance, and the product–moment correlation coefficient.

If you doubt whether to use a parametric statistical test with your data, consult a statistician. If told not to use parametrics, you need not despair. There are many suitable nonparametric tests, as will be shown below.

Table 4.2. *The use of chi-square (χ^2) and the phi coefficient (ϕ) in a two-fold table (data on mentally ill and normal primiparas who report that the woman's mother is dead)*

	Hospitalized psychiatric patients	Normal new mothers	Row totals
Mother dead	9	5	14
Mother alive	24	110	134
Total	33	115	148

$\chi^2 = 15.7$. $\phi = .326$. $p < .001$.

2. *Nonparametric.* These statistical tests may be used when the requirements of the parametrics cannot be met. Their difference from parametric statistics is that they are not based upon an assumption of a normally distributed population variable. They are not as powerful as the parametric tests, but they are easier to compute, and they will also allow you to make a probability statement about the significance of the group differences that you have found. Nonparametric tests include chi-square, the binomial test, the Wilcoxon matched-pairs signed-ranks test, the Spearman rank correlation coefficient, the phi coefficient, the contingency coefficient, and many others. Some are discussed below.

Examples of some simple nonparametrics and parametrics

Nonparametrics

Chi-square in a two-by-two table. Chi-square (χ^2) is a nonparametric statistic of association that may be used to calculate the significance of differences between groups or categories of populations measured by ordinal and nominal variables. It tests whether there is significant difference between an observed number of subjects or responses in a category and an expected number.

Table 4.2 uses χ^2 to measure differences between normal and hospitalized new mothers. It and Table 4.3 are adapted from data obtained in cross-validating the maternity questionnaire (Larsen et al., 1966). In Table 4.2, nine psychiatrically hospitalized women and five normal pri-

Table 4.3. *Occurrence of stressful events in the lives of psychiatrically hospitalized and normal new mothers*

	Percentage			Chi-square	
		Normals			
	Hospitalized (N = 33–34)	Primiparas (N = 103–127)	Triparas (N = 87–105)	Hospitalized vs. primiparas	Hospitalized vs. triparas
1. Interreligious marriage	32.2	6.6	12.1	***	*
2. Husband–wife conflict on women's role in family	20	1.9	3.4	**	*
3. No female relative nearby	74.1	92.8	26.9	**	***
4. Emotional difficulties in husband's family	45.1	13.9	7.1	***	**
5. Emotional difficulties in wife's family	66.6	17.7	20.6	***	***
6. Pregnancy complications in wife's family	48.2	22.5	25.0	*	*
7. Wife had emotional difficulties during this pregnancy	60.7	6.1	19.1	***	***
8. Husband not off work to help after birth of this baby	50.0	20.9	23.7	**	*
9. Husband plans no further education	45.1	6.9	75.0	*	**

10. Wife has had nonpregnant emotional problems	51.7	0	***	***
11. Wife has had nonpregnant physical problems	36.6	9.6	***	
12. Wife has had emotional difficulties with a previous pregnancy	32.0	0.8	***	**
13. Wife has had physical difficulties with a previous pregnancy	35.7	8.7	***	
14. Family made a major move of household during this pregnancy	48.3	29.5	***	***
15. Former marriage	30.3	2.7	***	
16. Wife's mother dead	27.2	4.3	***	
17. Wife's mother died before wife was 21 years	15.1	2.4	*	
18. Husband and wife out socially less than once a month	34.5	76.8	***	
19. Husband's father dead	40.0	16.1	**	
20. Husband's mother dead	24.1	7.3	*	
21. Husband has emotional difficulties	7.7	0	*	

The significance of these differences was calculated by chi-square. * Significant at the .05 level. ** Significant at the .01 level. *** Significant at the .001 level.

Source: Larsen et al., 1966.

miparas reported that the patient's mother was dead. This item is on a nominal scale, so χ^2 is the appropriate statistic. Note that Table 4.3 gives ranges for the total numbers of normal and hospitalized mothers. When filling out the questionnaire, a number of women did not answer certain items. When this occurs, present your findings in ranges, as shown in Table 4.3, but in your calculations use the actual numbers who checked an item. Table 4.2 indicates that 115 normal women filled in Item 16, as did 33 hospitalized women.

Table 4.2 is created by putting the numbers in a two-by-two matrix and summing the rows and the columns. Chapter 4.A shows how to perform the computations needed for the data in Table 4.2. Software packages exist for use with the home or office microcomputer that compute χ^2, but the computations for Table 4.2 are easily done in a few moments with the help of a hand calculator and a sheet of paper. Examples of the output of microcomputer programs appear in chapters 4.A and 5.A.

Performing repeated chi-squares on items within a test given to the same group of subjects is not an acceptable procedure for the final results of a study. In Table 4.3, the findings showed whether or not there were any important results. The researchers used repeated chi-squares in the case above to find out whether or not they were getting results similar to those we had reported. After seeing the striking results shown above, we subjected the data to an *item analysis* (see "Selecting Items" below). An item analysis is the appropriate method for determining the salient factors in a large group of test items.

Chi-square as a goodness-of-fit test. One of the most common uses of chi-square is to test how well a sample of data fits a known pattern or group of categories. For example, you might want to know if the prevalence of a specific emotional reaction is the same in all age groups or economic levels. Answering this question requires you to make a *goodness-of-fit* test; that is, you will test your obtained data against the expected frequencies in the pattern you have selected.

To make this comparison, use the formula $\chi^2 = \Sigma(o - e)^2/e$, where $o =$ the observed number of cases in a category,

$e =$ the expected number of cases in the same category, and

Σ means: Add all the $(o - e)^2/e$ quantities to obtain a single sum.

The data contained in Table 7.5 have been subjected to two chi-square goodness-of-fit tests. Note that one set of data is shown to fit a theoretical curve, but the other set of data does not fit the theoretical curve.

Probability of occurrence, significance, and degrees of freedom. The value of chi-square in Table 4.2 is 15.7. The probability (*p*) of this number occurring by chance is less than ($<$) 1 in 1,000 (.001), which is considered a *very highly significant* result (see chapter 4.A and Appendix Table A.1). The higher the χ^2 for any given degree of freedom, the greater its significance. Significance is generally presented as a decimal – .05 means 5% occurrence by chance, or *significant*; .01 means 1% occurrence by chance, or *highly significant*; .001 means 0.1% occurrence by chance, or *very highly significant*. The item above shows that women who became mentally ill and required hospitalization are very significantly more likely than normal primiparas to have lost their mothers.

The degrees of freedom are calculated by subtracting the number 1 from the number of rows (two in Table 4.2) and from the number of columns (again two), and multiplying the two difference numbers together: 1 times 1 equals one degree of freedom.

Chi-square is used as a statistic in over 8% of articles in the principal psychiatric journals (Hokanson et al., 1986). You choose it when:

1. You do not need the most sensitive analyses to prove your point
2. You do not have more precise ordinal, interval, or ratio-scaled numbers available
3. You want to obtain information quickly and easily about your data by hand calculation
4. You need a flexible statistic that can be applied to categorical data

For instance, suppose you wanted to determine whether two hospitals differed by age category in the numbers of patients treated over a period of time. You could obtain the numbers admitted to the hospitals in each of four groups – the children's, adolescents', adults', and geriatric programs. Then you could make a four-by-two table, and use χ^2 to calculate whether there was a difference between the two hospitals in the age categories of patients admitted. (However, if you wanted to obtain the difference between the hospitals by the mean age of all patients admitted, you would use a *t* test, as discussed below.)

You will often find chi-square used in the early stages of measurement, observed relation, observed causal, and causal relation research. You can calculate results by hand quickly with it and determine whether findings are statistically significant or not, and thus whether the research is worth pursuing. Certain correlations (defined below) can easily be obtained from χ^2, as will be shown later.

Correlation and phi coefficients. Correlation indicates the degree to which change in one variable is related to change in another. It provides a single number that summarizes the relationship between two variables. Correlations range from -1.0 for a perfect inverse relationship, where one variable gets larger as the other gets smaller, through 0, where there is no relationship at all, to $+1.0$ for a perfect positive relationship. The significance of a correlation is directly related to the sample size. The meaningfulness of the size of a correlation is related to the nature of the variable. For example, the correlation of a test with itself should be at least .90; on the other hand, the correlation of a measure like an I.Q. test with a criterion such as grade-point average is rarely more than .60; and interest tests correlate about .40 with behavior. Nevertheless, a good rule of thumb for relationships between most psychiatric variables is as follows: Correlations from .00 to .20 denote a negligible relationship; between .20 and .40, low to moderate; .40 to .60, moderate; .60 to .75, fairly strong; .75 to .85, strong; .85 and over, very strong.

The phi coefficient (ϕ) indicates the degree of association when the variables can be put into a two-by-two rows-by-columns table such as Table 4.2. It provides a nonparametric measure of correlation that can readily be calculated from χ^2. It is especially useful in item analyses of data such as those in Table 4.2, since it provides a measure of the relative importance of each item. It was used to give weights to the items in the maternity questionnaire discussed below. Instead of giving each significant item the same weight, we summed the ϕ values to provide a score on the questionnaire.

To calculate the phi coefficient (ϕ), divide chi-square ($\chi^2 = 15.7$) by the number of subjects ($N = 148$), and take the square root, as follows:

$$\phi = \sqrt{15.7/148} = .326.$$

The significance level of this low-to-moderate correlation is the same as that for its χ^2, $p < .001$.

Parametrics

Student's t test – the significance of the difference between two means. Student's *t* test is a parametric test. You use it when:

1. You have interval or ratio-scaled data
2. The observations are drawn from normally distributed populations;

Table 4.4. *Comparison of shorter-staying and longer-staying psychiatric inpatients by Axis IV and Axis V scores*

	No. patients	Axis IV score		Axis V score	
		Mean	*SD*	Mean	*SD*
<90-day inpatients	77	3.8	1.45	4.28	1.0
90+-day inpatients	149	4.5	1.16	5.0	.97

The differences are statistically significant. Comparing short-term inpatients and long-term inpatients by Axis IV, $t = 3.68$ and $p < .01$; by Axis V, $t = 5.14$ and $p < .01$.

the shape of their frequency distribution is like that of the normal curve shown in Figure 2.2

3. The variances of the population distributions of the two groups being examined are approximately equal

A cross-validation of the research on the usefulness of *DSM-III*'s new quantitative tests found that patients' Axis IV aggravating stress and Axis V premorbid functional level scores were related to the length of inpatient treatment they received, as shown in Table 4.4 (G. R. Zanni, personal communication, 1986). *DSM-III* treats Axes IV and V as interval scales. The researchers who collected the data shown in Table 4.4 reported the Axis IV and Axis V means and standard deviations for two groups of chronically ill longer- and shorter-staying psychiatric inpatients. These provide the data needed to show the procedure for calculating a *t* test.

The *t* value for the difference between the two mean Axis IV scores is 3.68 and between the two mean Axis V scores is 5.14. Chapter 4.A shows how to measure the significance of a difference between two means. Appendix Table A.2 provides the probabilities for different *t* values. The data provide support for other studies conducted with nonparametric statistics, which indicate that *DSM-III*'s quantitative scales may be valid measures that provide useful information in both clinical research and treatment (R. E. Gordon & Gordon, 1987).

The *t* test described above is a *two-tailed* t test and therefore answers only the question "Is there a significant difference?" When attempting to answer statistically a question about whether or not a specified mean is significantly larger than or significantly smaller than another specified mean, a one-tailed *t* test must be used. The distinction will not be explored here; the reader is referred to Runyon (1985), where it is discussed fully.

The t test is employed in 10% of the articles in the major psychiatric journals (Hokanson et al., 1986). It takes more time to perform by hand the arithmetic computations needed in a t test than those in a chi-square analysis, especially if you are dealing with more than 10 cases. However, you need not go through these steps nowadays to analyze your data. Computer programs exist for both mainframe and personal microcomputers that calculate all these and other more complicated parametric and non-parametric statistics, including the multivariate statistics discussed in the next chapter.

Presenting data in tables

Tables 4.2 and 4.3 contain large amounts of information in condensed form. Table 4.3, like many others in the psychiatric literature, uses percentages to compare findings between groups, presents chi-squares for each pair of compared data, and shows the significance level by means of asterisks. The meanings of the asterisks appear in the table notes. The data in Table 4.3 show that a number of stressful events occur with greater frequency in the lives of hospitalized maternity psychiatric patients than in the lives of normal new mothers.

Table 4.4 presents its data with the variables' means, standard deviations, and t tests.

In preparing a table, make certain that your column and row headings clearly label the data so that your readers can easily understand what they are reading, and that your notes or text explain what you found. It is a good idea to show your tables to colleagues, perhaps in a staff presentation, before you submit them to publishers in order to determine whether you have accomplished these goals. Some of the computer software for statistical analyses on the microcomputer produce attractive tables and graphs for displaying data and statistical analyses that can be printed and submitted for publication.

Creating a new questionnaire

The developers of the psychiatric tests and rating scales described earlier in this chapter have gone through all the steps that follow, and more. However, few practicing clinical psychiatrists will wish to undertake the lengthy process of developing and standardizing a psychosocial questionnaire. But you should know what is involved so that you can evaluate the usefulness of an instrument you are considering and determine whether it meets your needs.

The principles discussed here also apply to the patient history and data-collection forms you may use for patient assessment and evaluation purposes with your own patients. In many new research areas, there may be no adequate questionnaire or rating scale. Then you may need to develop your own tool, probably with the help of an expert. However, your clinical experience and hunches from patients in your practice will help you in selecting a group of initial items for the clinical test, as shown in the next sections.

The development of the maternity questionnaire illustrates how questionnaires and other clinical test instruments and scales are created. The questionnaire was put together with social history items obtained from treating our psychiatric and other maternity patients. It was not intended for general use as a clinical rating scale like the instruments discussed earlier. Instead, it was developed as part of our psychiatric maternity research. It helped to identify and score the kinds of stresses with which perinatal women were coping, to assess their needs, to select patients for correlational and experimental studies, and to determine population norms. In many respects it was a kind of data-collection form, similar to those discussed previously, which obtain a great deal of information about each patient in a systematic way. The steps involved in its development include *selecting and analyzing items* and *determining reliability and validity*.

Selecting items

In constructing a clinical test or instrument, you must first develop a battery of items that individually discriminate significantly between your research group and normals or others with whom you wish to make comparisons. Each item should clearly address a single question. You should avoid loading your questions in a manner that would bias the patients' or other subjects' responses. Likewise, if your questions call for *agree* or *disagree* answers, do not ask them in a way that leads a person with a certain attitude to give all *agree* or all *disagree* responses. If you do, persons answering the questions will begin to respond automatically, without giving thought to their answers. Instead, phrase half of them so that responders will agree with them, and phrase the other half so they will disagree. And scatter the agree/disagree questions randomly through the

Table 4.5. *Items from an early draft of the maternity stress questionnaire (illustrates an instrument difficult for both patient and researcher to score)*

Where do you live?   Own home   Apartment   Someone else's home
Who lives with you besides husband and children? _____ _____
  Is he or she in good health?   Yes   No
Who of wife's other relatives live in Bergen County?
  Mother   Father   Sister   Brother   None
Who of husband's other relatives live in Bergen County?
  Mother   Father   Sister   Brother   None
In how many towns did wife live before she was eighteen? _____
In how many towns did husband live before he was eighteen? _____
In how many towns has couple lived since marriage? _____
How many close friends with babies or young children does wife have?
  None   1   2   3   4   5   More
How many of your neighbors have babies or young children?
  None   1   2   3   4   5   More
Is wife trying to make more friends with babies or young children?   Yes   No

6. Transportation: How many cars do wife and husband own?   None   One   More
  Do you live within five blocks of a bus station?   Yes   No
  Does wife drive?   Yes   No   Does she plan driving lessons?   Yes   No   When? _____

7. Family Medical History
Has anyone in husband's family ever had a problem with drinking or an emotional difficulty?   Yes   No
  Who? _____   What was   Nothing   Hospitalized   Saw a psychiatrist   Other
  _____   done a-   Nothing   Hospitalized   Saw a psychiatrist   Other
  _____   bout it?   Nothing   Hospitalized   Saw a psychiatrist   Other
Has anyone in wife's family ever had a problem with drinking or an emotional difficulty?   Yes   No
  Who? _____   What was   Nothing   Hospitalized   Saw a psychiatrist   Other
  _____   done a-   Nothing   Hospitalized   Saw a psychiatrist   Other
  _____   bout it?   Nothing   Hospitalized   Saw a psychiatrist   Other
Did anyone in wife's family have complications of pregnancy or childbearing?
  Physical complications   Yes   No
  Who? _____   What compli- _____   Hospitalized?   Yes   No
  _____   cation?   _____   Yes   No
  _____   _____   Yes   No
  Emotional complications: Yes   No
  Who? _____   What compli- _____   Hospitalized?   Yes   No
  _____   cation?   _____   Yes   No
  _____   _____   Yes   No
Have either of husband's parents died?   Yes   No
  Who? _____   When? _____   At what age? _____   How old was husband? _____
Have either of wife's parents died?   Yes   No
  Who? _____   When? _____   At what age? _____   How old was wife? _____
Did husband's parents ever separate?   Yes   No
  Why?   They couldn't get along   Because of work or war   How old was he? _____
Did wife's parents ever separate?   Yes   No
  Why?   They couldn't get along   Because of work or war   How old was she? _____

8. Personal Medical History
Menses: Age of onset: _____   Regular   Irregular   How many days of flow? _____
How many days between periods? _____   Discomfort: Much   Some   Little
Serious physical illness of wife   Yes   No   At what age? _____
  Describe _____   Hospitalized?   Yes   No   Operation?   Yes   No
  _____   Yes   No   Yes   No

questionnaire, so that there is no special section with questions that responders are sure to answer one way.

The maternity questionnaire sought to determine how psychiatric maternity patients differed in their social backgrounds from emotionally normal new mothers. Life-history items in the lives of two groups of women were compared. The first was a sample of 55 psychiatric maternity patients treated in office practice; the other, 98 normal maternity patients residing on the obstetrical unit of the local general hospital after delivering normal babies. The first draft of the maternity questionnaire contained stress-related items that were occurring with greater frequency in the lives of maternity psychiatric patients. A page from this early questionnaire appears in Table 4.5. These items included events like wife's mother's death. Chi-square tests of differences identified the 21 items shown earlier in Table 4.3.

This form of the maternity questionnaire is far from ideal. It presents problems for the person filling it in and for the person interpreting the responses. A subsequent modification of the instrument, shown in Table 4.6, is more suitable for use with a computer. Comparing the two, you can see how difficult and time-consuming it would be both to fill in and to analyze the items in Table 4.5 as compared with those in Table 4.6. The second form is explicit and provides a numerical code for each response. Every response in the first would need to be coded before data could be pooled and analyzed.

Next, you must determine whether your collection of items discriminates significantly between research groups and normals. We and other researchers administered this draft questionnaire to a number of groups of maternity psychiatric patients and normals. Table 4.3 shows comparative results obtained with three populations of maternity patients – hospitalized psychiatric patients, normal triparas, and normal primiparas – who filled in the questionnaire. Clearly, the women's questionnaire responses indicate that each of these stressful events occurred to a greater extent in the lives of psychiatric maternity patients than in those of normal new mothers.

A next step – item analysis – is beyond the scope of this book; it is mentioned here so that you will be familiar with the process. Since many psychosocial items (and chemical and physiological tests, too) measure the same thing, they duplicate each other. It is wasteful of time and money repeatedly to obtain the same information in assessing a patient. It is therefore necessary to identify and weed out duplicative measures and to put them aside. They can be used, however, to create an alternate form of a clinical test. You can use an alternate form when you wish to retest patients after they have undergone some treatment, and are con-

Table 4.6. *Items from a later draft of the maternity stress questionnaire (illustrates an instrument more suitable for patients to fill in and computers to analyze)*

20. My Family Problems:
    0 – None of my family have had nervous difficulties or problems with alcohol or drugs.
        1 – One or more members of my family have had nervous difficulties or problems with alcohol or drugs.
        Who? _____

        _____

21. Husband's Family Problems:
    0 – None of his family have had nervous difficulties or problems with alcohol or drugs.
        1 – One or more members of his family have had nervous difficulties or problems with alcohol or drugs.
        Who? _____

        _____

22. My Parents' Marriage:
    0 – My parents have had a happy marriage
        1 – My parents did not have a happy marriage, but did not separate or divorce
        2 – My parents are separated or divorced.
23. Husband's Parents' Marriage:
    0 – His parents did not have a happy marriage.
        1 – His parents did not have a happy marriage, but did not separate or divorce.
        2 – His parents are separated or divorced.
24. My Mother's Health:
    0 – My mother is living.
        1 – My mother died before I was 12 years old.
        2 – My mother died after I was 12, but before I was 21.
        3 – My mother died after I was 21.
25. My Father's Health:
    0 – My father is living.
        1 – My father died before I was 12 years old.
        2 – My father died after I was 12, but before I was 21.
        3 – My father died after I was 21.
26. Husband's Mother's Health:
    0 – My husband's mother is living.
        1 – My husband's mother died before he was 12 years old.
        2 – My husband's mother died after he was 12, but before he was 21.
        3 – My husband's mother died after he was 21.

Table 4.7. *The use of chi-square (χ^2) and the contingency coefficient (C) in a two-by-three table (compares ratings of maternity patients' postpartum emotional reaction and their scores on the maternity stress questionnaire)*

No. of stressful items on questionnaire	No. of patients with this number of stresses	No. and % of patients rated emotionally			
		Normal		Distressed	
		No.	%	No.	%
0–2	90	85	94.4	5	5.6
3–4	71	50	70.4	21	29.6
5 or more	46	18	39.1	28	60.9
Total no. of patients	207	153		54	

$\chi^2 = 48.99.$ $df = 2.$ $C = .437$ $(C_{max} = .816).$ $p < .001.$

cerned that their having taken the same form of the test previously may influence their responses on retesting.

Validity of the questionnaire

To determine whether a questionnaire does what it is intended to do, you must measure its validity.

The maternity questionnaire was used to select women who were at high risk for postpartum emotional distress. It was administered to 207 recently delivered mothers on the obstetrical ward. Two months later, their obstetricians rated the severity of the patients' postpartum emotional distress. Table 4.7 presents their ratings (R. E. Gordon, 1961). These findings indicate that the maternity questionnaire has a good degree of validity and is potentially useful for predicting postpartum emotional distress.

Another study showed that the correlation was .69 between questionnaire scores and those on a psychiatric symptom scale administered during pregnancy, and was .49 with the score on the symptom scale when it was administered in the first trimester after delivery (see chapter 5). These findings serve to cross-validate those reported in Table 4.7.

Another statistic: the contingency coefficient

Table 4.7 is a two-by-three table. Tables of this size and larger require a different approach to calculating χ^2 than that for a two-by-two table. Table 4.7 also uses C – the *contingency coefficient* – to show the correlation between ratings of maternity patients' postpartum emotional reaction and their scores on the maternity questionnaire. Chapter 4.A shows how to calculate χ^2 in two-by-three and larger tables.

The contingency coefficient is used like the phi coefficient to measure correlation with nonparametric variables, those with ordinal or nominal scales. Like the phi coefficient, the contingency coefficient can easily be computed from chi-square. Its formula is:

$$C = \sqrt{\frac{\chi^2}{N + \chi^2}} = \sqrt{\frac{49}{207 + 49}} = \sqrt{\frac{49}{256}} = .437$$

Use C when a table contains more than two rows or columns, as in Table 4.7, where there are two rows by three columns. (When there are exactly two rows and two columns, use the phi coefficient.)

A disadvantage of C is that it does not remain constant for the same data when the number of classes varies. Furthermore, the maximum value that C can take depends upon the fineness of the classification used. The maximum value increases as the number of classes increases, ranging up from a (C_{max}) of .707 when the number of classes is only 2 to a C_{max} of .949 when the number of classes is 10.

Reliability of the questionnaire

When measurement of validity depends upon human judgments, as in the example above, where obstetricians assessed the emotional reactions of maternity patients, the reliability of the judges also needs to be determined.

The reliability of the obstetricians' ratings of 214 maternity patients was obtained by having each patient rated twice. This was done either by having two different doctors rate the same patient or by having the same doctor rate the patient at two different times. Then the first set of ratings on each patient was correlated with the second set. The correlation between the two independent sets of judgments was .86 (R. E. Gordon, 1961), which is quite acceptable.

Sensitivity and specificity

If you employ a clinical test to help diagnose a disease, you will be interested in its sensitivity and specificity. Sensitivity refers to the test's ability to diagnose the presence of the disease in patients who actually have it. Mathematically, it is the number of positive findings obtained by a test divided by the total number of true positives.

In the context used here, specificity is the opposite of sensitivity. It refers to the test's ability to confirm the absence of disease in patients who do not have it. It is measured by the number of negative findings divided by the total number of negatives.

Obtaining norms

The maternity questionnaire provided an instrument that helped identify patients for both correlational and experimental studies. It served to identify and score the same standard information on the kinds and amounts of stresses with which maternity patients were coping.

And it served another valuable purpose: It was used periodically to collect social histories from sequential samples of normal women who were delivering their babies at our community hospital. This information on ages of women and their husbands, their religions, numbers of children, lengths of stay in the community, and so on was useful data about this population group in the community. The information provided comparison data for research studies that showed how patient groups differed from their normal counterparts in the community.

Comment on creating a new instrument

Since the maternity questionnaire showed that stressful life events could be used as items in a quantitative measure, it helped spur the development of more comprehensive and widely used instruments like the well-known Holmes and Rahe Social Adjustment Rating Scale (Holmes & Rahe, 1967) and the Axis IV aggravating stress scale of *DSM-III*. Instruments like the maternity questionnaire that focus on experiences related to a specific life role – early motherhood – have limited value in comparison with those like the Holmes and Rahe scale and Axis IV. The Holmes and Rahe scale provides a simple, standardized, and relatively comprehensive general measure of stress caused by a variety of life events that affect everyone, regardless of age, sex, or demographics. The maternity questionnaire pays attention to specific stresses – background sensitizers, ongoing pressurizers, and present-day precipitators – that impair the functioning of pregnant women and young mothers.

Research with these scales and others like them that measure stress has repeatedly shown the relationship between aggravating stress and physical and psychiatric illness. They have contributed to the development of a psychiatric law: *Stress can lead to distress.*

Operationally, amount of stress is defined as a score on a stress instrument such as the Axis IV scale, and amount of distress is defined as the score on a scale such as the one obstetricians used to rate their patients' postpartum emotional reactions.

Summary

Chapter 4 has described measurement research and explained how and why researchers should plan their research before beginning to collect data. It introduces the subject of random selection, defines the role of statistics in research, and discusses types of statistics (parametric and nonparametric), types of measurement (nominal, ordinal, interval, and ratio scales), and types of variables (discrete and continuous). It shows how the statistic or statistical test chosen depends upon the types of variables and types of measurements.

As examples of measurement research, the chapter describes some work that attempts to determine whether the two quantitative scales of *DSM-III,* the Axis IV aggravating stress scale and the Axis V premorbid functional level scale, are valid and useful. It discusses standardized psychiatric tests and rating scales and illustrates the creation of a questionnaire, the maternity questionnaire. Finally, it presents some examples of the use of chi-square (χ^2), some other nonparametric statistics, and Student's *t* test.

Chapter 4.A shows how to calculate some of these statistics.

4.A. Simple statistics

Nonparametric statistics

Calculating chi-square in two-by-two contingency tables

Chi-square (χ^2) compares observed frequencies with expected frequencies. If the ratio of the former to the latter exceeds certain values (which are shown in Appendix A.1), the difference is significant. We shall use the data in Table 4.2 to show how to calculate χ^2 in a two-by-two table. Notice that in Table 4.2 and in Table 4.3, Item 16, 27.2% (9 persons) of 33 psychiatrically hospitalized women and 4.3% (5 persons) of 115 normal primiparas reported that the wife's mother was dead. To calculate the significance of the difference between the responses to this item by hospitalized and normal women, create a two-by-two table. Put in the sums of the actual numbers of women who responded in the rows and columns and calculate as follows in Table 4.A.1.

Turning to Appendix Table A.1, the chi-square table, we select the row that corresponds to the degree of freedom in our table. Degrees of freedom for chi-square tables are calculated by subtracting the number 1 from the number of rows (two in Table 4.A.1) and from the number of columns (also two), and multiplying the two difference numbers: 1 times 1 equals 1 degree of freedom (*df*). We find that for 1 *df* the value 15.7 is highly significant. The probability that it could have occurred by chance is less than 1 in 1,000 trials ($p < .001$). Generally, the larger a χ^2 for a given *df*, the greater the likelihood that the observed frequencies did not come from the population on which the bulk hypothesis was based.

Using phi coefficients as measures of correlation

Phi coefficients (ϕ) are used to indicate the degree of association when a variable can be put into a two-by-two rows-by-columns table such as that

83

Table 4.A.1. *The calculation of chi-square in a two-by-two table*

Row 1	9 (A)	5 (B)	14 (A + B)
Row 2	24 (C)	110 (D)	134 (C + D)
Total	33	115	148
	(A + C)	(B + D)	(A + B + C + D)

Calculate x^2 from the formula:

$$x^2 = \frac{(A + B + C + D)(AD - BC)^2}{(A + B)(C + D)(A + C)(B + D)}$$

Substituting in the formula,

$$x^2 = \frac{148 \times 870 \times 870}{14 \times 134 \times 33 \times 115} = 15.7$$

in 4.A.1. To calculate the phi coefficient, divide x^2 by the number of subjects ($N = 148$ in Table 4.A.1), and take the square root, as follows:

$$\phi = \sqrt{15.7/148} = .326$$

The significance of this modest correlation is the same as that for its $x^2 - p < .001$. Thus, in Table 4.2, the three values at the bottom of the table – $x^2 = 15.7$; $\phi = .326$; $p < .001$ – tell us the value of chi-square, its related phi coefficient, and its probability of occurrence by chance. This is the standard way in which these data are presented in scientific tables in the medical literature.

Table 4.A.2 presents the results of a computer analysis of the data in Tables 4.2 and 4.A.1, providing the x^2, ϕ, and another statistic that will be discussed later – the contingency coefficient. We conducted this analysis and other statistical tests in this book on a Macintosh microcomputer with the StatView™ program (Feldman & Gagnon, 1985), which cost only $44.

Calculating chi-square in two-by-three and larger tables

In the example in Table 4.A.1 we calculated x^2 from data in a two-by-two table. The procedure is different, but still quite simple, for computing x^2 with two-by-three and larger tables. In Table 4.7, a two-by-three table compares ratings of maternity patients' postpartum emotional reaction with their scores on the maternity questionnaire. To calculate x^2, obtain

Table 4.A.2. *A microcomputer analysis of the data in Table 4.A.1*

Contingency Table Analysis	
Summary Statistics	
DF:	1
Total Chi-Square:	15.735 p ≤ .001
G Statistic:	12.853
Contingency Coefficient:	.31
Phi:	.326
Chi-Square with continuity correction:	13.172 p ≤ .001

1

Contingency Table Analysis

	Column #1	Column #2	Totals:
Row #1	9	5	14
	R%: 64.29	R%: 35.71	9.46%
	C%: 27.27	C%: 4.35	
Row #2	24	110	134
	R%: 17.91	R%: 82.09	90.54%
	C%: 72.73	C%: 95.65	
Totals:	33	115	148
	22.3%	77.7%	

2

the sums of the rows and columns, as shown here in Table 4.A.3 in arabic numerals. Then compute each row total's percentage of the whole group by dividing it by the group N, and place its value in parentheses in the far right-hand column as shown. Now calculate the expected values for each cell by multiplying each of the two column totals for the two patient groups by the percentages in the right-hand column, as follows: $153 \times .222 = 34$; $153 \times .343 = 52.5$; $153 \times .435 = 66.6$; $54 \times .222 =$

Table 4.A.3. *The calculation of chi-square in two-by-three and larger tables*

	Observed no.	(Expected no.)	Observed no.	(Expected no.)	
Row 1	85	(66.6)	5	(23.5)	90 (90/207) = (.435)
Row 2	50	(52.5)	21	(18.4)	71 (71/207) = (.343)
Row 3	18	(.34)	28	(12.0)	46 (46/207) = (.222)
Total	153		54		207

$$85 - 66.6 = 18.4; 18.4 \times 18.4/66.6 = 5.080$$
$$52.5 - 50 = 2.5; 2.5 \times 2.5/52.5 = 0.119$$
$$34 - 18 = 16; 16 \times 16/34 = 7.529$$
$$23.5 - 5 = 18.5; 18.5 \times 18.5/23.5 = 14.564$$
$$21 - 18.4 = 2.6; 2.6 \times 2.6/18.4 = 0.368$$
$$28 - 12 = 16; 16 \times 16/12 = 21.333$$

Summing these figures, we get 48.993, or about 49.0, which is the value of chi-square (χ^2)

12; $54 \times .343 = 18.4$; $54 \times .435 = 23.5$. Place these numbers in the appropriate cells above in italics and parentheses.

Next, calculate for each cell entry the difference between the observed and the expected number, square the difference number, and divide the squared result by the expected number, as shown in Table 4.A.3.

From Appendix Table A.1, row 2 for 2 degrees of freedom (df), we learn that a value of 49 or greater could have occurred by chance less than once in 1,000 trials ($p < .001$). (Actually, the value 49 could have occurred by chance less than once in 10,000 – $p = <.0001$ – but most tables do not provide values beyond the .001 level.) We calculated the degrees of freedom, as before, by subtracting 1 from the number of rows ($3 - 1 = 2$), and 1 from the number of columns ($2 - 1 = 1$) and multiplying the products ($2 \times 1 = 2$).

Table 4.A.4 shows a computer analysis of the data in Tables 4.7 and 4.A.3, again providing χ^2, ϕ, and the contingency coefficient.

Generally, you can use χ^2 when fewer than 20% of the cells have an expected frequency of 5 or less. When you find that this will be a problem, you can frequently collapse your data into a smaller number of rows and columns and thus into fewer cells. This was done in computing the χ^2 in Table 7.5, where the number of cells was decreased from 10 to 6. No cells now have an expected frequency of less than 5.

Table 4.A.4. *A microcomputer analysis of data in Table 4.A.3*

Contingency Table Analysis

Summary Statistics

DF:	2
Total Chi-Square:	48.987 p ≤ .001
G Statistic:	51.194
Contingency Coefficient:	.437
Cramer's V:	.486

1

Contingency Table Analysis

	Column #1	Column #2	Totals:
Row #1	85 R%: 94.44 C%: 55.56	5 R%: 5.56 C%: 9.26	90 43.48%
Row #2	50 R%: 70.42 C%: 32.68	21 R%: 29.58 C%: 38.89	71 34.3%
Row #3	18 R%: 39.13 C%: 11.76	28 R%: 60.87 C%: 51.85	46 22.22%
Totals:	153 73.91%	54 26.09%	207

2

Table 4.A.5. *The calculation of chi-square when cell entries for expected values are less than 5, with Yates's correction for continuity applied*

	Hospitalized		Normal primipara		Row totals	
	Observed	(Expected)	Observed	(Expected)		
Previous pregnancy emotional difficulties	11	(2.55)	1	(9.45)	12	(.075)
No previous pregnancy emotional difficulties	23	(31.45)	125	(116.55)	148	(.925)
Column totals	34		126		160	

In calculating χ^2 we decrease the absolute value of the difference between the obtained and expected values in each cell by 0.5. The difference between 11 and 2.55, 23 and 31.45, 1 and 9.45, and 125 and 116.55 (= 8.45) is reduced to 7.95. Then the calculations proceed as shown in Table 4.A.2:

$$7.95^2/2.55 = 24.8; \ 7.95^2/31.45 = 2.01; \ 7.95^2/9.45 = 6.69, \ \text{and} \ 7.95^2/116.55 = 0.54.$$

Summing, we get $\chi^2 = 34.0$. Appendix Table A.1 shows that this value is significant beyond the .001 level for 1 df.

Calculating chi-square with expected frequencies containing fewer than five members

Take a look now at Table 4.3, Item 12, "Wife has had emotional difficulties with a previous pregnancy." Among women who required psychiatric hospitalization, this event occurred in the lives of 11 (32%) of 34 women. However, only 1 (0.8%) of 126 normal women had had emotional difficulties in a previous pregnancy. We set up Table 4.A.5 in the same manner as we did Table 4.A.3. Note that there is an expected value of 2.55. But χ^2 is not stable when computed from a two-by-two table in which any expected value is less than 5. Therefore in calculating χ^2 we use *Yates's correction for continuity.*

Obtaining the contingency coefficient (C) from chi-square

To obtain the contingency coefficient (C) from chi-square in Table 4.A.3, we divide chi-square by the sum of chi-square plus the number of subjects, and obtain the square root of the quotient as follows:

$$C = \sqrt{49/(49 + 207)} = \sqrt{49/256} = \sqrt{.19} = .437.$$

Note that the microcomputer output in Table 4.A.4 provides this contingency coefficient.

Parametric statistics

Calculating the standard deviation (SD)

The standard deviation and mean are used in parametric statistics. To compute the *SD* you obtain each of the deviations of the measures from the group mean; then you square each deviation *(Dev)* and find their sum. You divide the sum by the total number of scores. Finally, you obtain the square root of this number. In mathematical terms the formula for the *SD* is as follows:

$$SD = \sqrt{\Sigma Dev^2 / N}$$

where *Dev* means each deviation, sigma (Σ) means the sum, and N refers to the total number of scores. The *SD* for a normally distributed variable often can be roughly estimated by taking one-fourth of the range. The range is defined as the difference between the largest and smallest mea-

Table 4.A.6. *The calculation of the standard deviation*

Football player	Uric acid level	Dev	Dev²
A	6	1	1
B	4	−1	1
C	3	−2	4
D	7	2	4
E	5	0	0
F	7	2	4
G	3	2	4
H	6	1	1
I	4	1	1
J	5	0	0
Total	50		20

M (mean) = 50/10 = 5

$N = 10$, $N - 1 = 9$ Sum of $Dev^2 = 20$
$SD = \sqrt{\Sigma Dev^2/(N - 1)} = \sqrt{20/9} = 1.49$

surements. (This is from a minus to a plus infinity for a normal distribution if you refer to population.) When the size of the sample is small (i.e., under 20), as in the example that follows, you must use the formula $SD = \sqrt{\Sigma Dev^2/(N - 1)}$.

Table 4.A.6 shows a selected group of 10 college football players' spring serum uric acid levels. (These are artificial data rounded out to whole numbers for ease of computation in the illustration.) Table 4.A.6 demonstrates how to calculate the standard deviation when the number of subjects is small.

When you have 20 or more subjects, it is a waste of time to go through all of the repetitious steps involved in obtaining and squaring the deviations and doing the other calculations, since many programs for personal minicomputers are now available to carry out these procedures for you. All you need to do is plug in the values and let the computer perform the chores.

Table 4.A.7 shows the output from a StatView program for data obtained from Table 4.A.6. Note that it includes the mean, standard deviation, and many other statistics, some of which are not discussed in this book.

Table 4.A.7. *A microcomputer analysis of the data in Table 4.A.6, providing mean, standard deviation, and many other statistics*

		Uric Acid Level				
Mean:	Std. Dev.:	Std. Error:	Variance:	Coef. Var.:	Count:	
5	1.491	.471	2.222	29.814	10	
Minimum:	Maximum:	Range:	Sum:	Sum Squared:	* Missing:	
3	7	4	50	270	0	

Table 4.A.8. *The use of the* t *test to calculate the significance of the difference between two means*

$$Dif = M_2 - M_1 = 4.5 - 3.8 = 0.7$$
$$SE_{M1} = SD_1/\sqrt{N_1} = 1.45/\sqrt{77} = 1.45/8.77 = 0.165$$
$$SE_{M2} = SD_2/\sqrt{N_2} = 1.16/\sqrt{149} = 1.16/12.2 = 0.095$$
$$SE_{Dif} = \sqrt{(SE_{M1})^2 + (SE_{M2})^2} = \sqrt{0.165^2 + 0.0975^2} = 0.19$$
$$t = Dif/SE_{Dif} = 0.7/0.19 = 3.68$$

To obtain the significance level of this t value, look at Appendix Table A.2. To determine the degrees of freedom (df) in this t test, subtract 1 from N_1 $(77 - 1 = 76)$, and 1 from N_2 $(149 - 1 = 148)$, and add the two numbers $(76 + 148 = 224)$. In column 1 for df, the number 224 comes between the last and next-to-last rows of the table. In the next-to-last row, the value of 3.68 is larger than the number 3.37 in the farthest right-hand column, for the 0.001 level of probability. Therefore this t value could not have occurred by chance more than once in 1,000 times.

Measuring the significance of a difference between two means

To measure the significance of a difference between two groups of scores on an equal-interval or a ratio scale, you compute a t test. The formula for t is

$$t = \text{Difference } (Dif)/\text{standard error of } Dif$$

where Dif is the difference between the two independent means. To obtain the standard error (SE) of Dif you first divide each mean's standard deviation by the square root of its N to obtain the SE of each mean, where N is the number of subjects. Then you square the two SEs of each mean, sum them, and obtain the square root of their sum.

As an example of this calculation, take the data from Table 4.4 on the difference between the Axis IV scores of patients who stayed in the hos-

Table 4.A.9a. *A microcomputer-generated table for comparing the progress of a group of patients after a year of treatment (data from Table 8.10)*

	Initial Current Axis U Score X	Current Axis U Score After One Year Y	Difference
1	6.0	4.4	1.6
2	5.3	2.4	2.9
3	5.5	3.4	2.1
4	6.4	5.0	1.4
5	5.2	3.8	1.4
6	6.2	4.8	1.4
7	6.0	3.0	3.0
8	5.4	4.3	1.1
9	5.3	2.8	2.5
10	6.2	3.0	3.2

Table 4.A.9b. *A* t-*test output from a microcomputer analysis (data from Tables 4.A.9a and 8.10)*

Paired t-Test X : Initial Current Axis V Score   Y : Current Axis V Score After One Year

DF:	Mean X – Y:	Paired t value:
9	2.06	8.315

p ≤ .0005

pital fewer than 90 days (mean $[M_1]$ = 3.8, standard deviation $[SD_1]$ = 1.45, number of subjects $[N_1]$ = 77) and scores of patients who remained 90 days or longer (mean $[M_2]$ = 4.5, standard deviation $[SD_2]$ = 1.16, number of subjects $[N_2]$ = 149). The calculations are shown in Table 4.A.8.

A StatView computerized analysis of the scores and *t* test shown in Table 8.10 appears in Tables 4.A.9a and b. Tables 8.10 and 4.A.9a show initial and subsequent scores of 10 patients whose progress in treatment was measured with the Axis V scale used to assess current functional level.

5. Observed relation research

Observed relation research, otherwise known as correlational research, is common yet often misunderstood. Some researchers and laymen tend to confuse correlation with cause. The discussions that follow address this problem but do not repeat aspects of research steps discussed in previous chapters. Those steps continue to apply here.

Definition

A research has reached the observed relation stage if it fulfills the following criteria:

1. There are two or more measurements on each of at least two measured variables
2. Changes in one variable are related to (but do not necessarily cause) changes in the other
3. Other factors (known or unknown) may or may not be held constant

The preceding chapter dealt with measurement research, in which you determine how to measure a variable. Observed relation research ranks a step higher. When you have measured two variables in two independent batches of data, you can now test the hypothesis that there is a relationship between the variables. Take a random sample from each batch, and calculate the correlation. The essential difference between this procedure and an experiment is that you impose no changes on the situation, but examine only the existing state of affairs. You thus determine whether the concepts are related to each other. No matter how large or statistically significant the correlation, you may not infer causality from an observed relation. You may not say whether increases in the first variable caused changes in the value of the second, or whether changes in the second caused changes in the first, or whether other unmeasured factors were

Table 5.1. *Assessing community psychiatric needs: observed relations between mean Axis IV scores, Axis V scores, and strain ratios of patients in three community treatment settings*

Outpatients	Growth of community	No. of patients	Mean Axis IV score	Mean Axis V score	Mean strain ratio[a]
Collier Co.	27%	55	4.8	3.6	1.3
Lee Co.	22.7%	124	4.5	3.7	1.2
Alachua Co.	11.1%	442	3.9	4.1	0.9

[a]In order to calculate the strain ratio, Axis V scores have been reversed in direction by subtracting the raw score from the number 8. As a result, high Axis V scores mean better levels of functioning, and lower scores worse.

The differences among the Axis IV scores, Axis V scores, and *SR*s are significant statistically (p ranged from .02 to .001).

responsible for the changes. However, findings from observed relation research may lead to causal relation experiments, as will be discussed in later chapters.

Many hypotheses about relationships between symptoms and diagnoses, stress and dysfunction, metabolic patterns and disorder, or between brain images and diseases are derived from observed relationships. You may first suspect a relationship in clinical practice in the form of a subtle trend or impression. A diagnosis can be regarded as a correlate of life events, symptoms, test results, or other clinical findings.

Making an observed relation hypothesis

Once you have established the validity and reliability of a measure, you may want to use it in observed relationship studies. For example, we first examined the validity of *DSM-III*'s two quantitative scales – Axis IV (aggravating stress) and Axis V (premorbid functional level). *DSM-III* presented measures of their reliability. Now we were ready to look at these two concepts in observed relation studies. Table 5.1 presents Axes IV and V scores and strain ratios (*SR*s) of patients from three different communities with different rates of growth (R. E. Gordon & Gordon, 1987). It uses the *DSM-III* measures to test the hypothesis that there is a relationship between social mobility and psychiatric disorder.

The fastest growing area – Collier County in southwestern Florida – grew 27% by immigration from out of state from 1980 to 1984 (see Table 5.1). Lee County's growth rate was 22.7%, and Alachua County's was 11.1%. The table compares the three communities' mean Axis IV and Axis V scores. It also looks at the ratio of Axis IV (aggravating stress) to Axis V (premorbid functional level), the strain ratio (*SR*) in each community. Table 5.1 shows that there was a perfect correspondence between community growth rate, Axis IV score, Axis V score, and strain ratio.

Deciding on subjects/patients

The hospital and office as clinical laboratories

You can easily and cheaply perform a retrospective review of patient records to test a hypothesis. A retrospective study is one in which an action has already occurred and been recorded. You merely go back to the records and look at what happened, as we did to obtain the data for Table 5.1.

The data in Table 5.1 came from outpatient records in three outpatient clinics in three areas. The research cost only the price of one overnight motel bill and driving to the clinics. Had the records been computerized, as is now the case in many facilities, we would have needed but a few telephone calls to obtain the data with a microcomputer and modem without leaving our office.

It costs even less to study your own practice. First, you need a well-designed standardized intake questionnaire or data-collection form that systematically records the information you want on all your patients. Then you can store the information in a personal computer for later retrieval and analysis. You, your office assistant, the patients themselves, or all three can fill in the data form. Later you can perform any of the kinds of research discussed in this book either by hand calculator or with the help of a computer.

Public appeals

You can also obtain data by appealing to the public for information. To launch the study *Rape and Its Victims,* the local media were asked to publicize our need for volunteers who had been rape victims. We wanted to find out where, when, and to whom such attacks had occurred, and whether and how such attacks had been warded off. Newspaper, radio, and television personnel provided excellent cooperation. This chapter discusses some of the findings.

Deciding on test instruments

Often clinicians will fortuitously be in a position to try out new test instruments that become available to them in their own clinical practices. In recent years brain imaging devices have become available. They have made possible many studies of the biological concomitants of mental disorders.

When autoanalyzers first became available to measure serum chemical levels, we were working part time on a college campus, both providing psychiatric treatment services and conducting observed relation studies. The latter were part of a program of needs assessments aimed at determining what students needed to know in order to succeed academically and to avoid health and disciplinary problems. The information was used in a program to orient students to college (Lindeman, Gordon & Gordon, 1969).

It cost little to obtain serum chemical data on students. Furthermore, with their grades, Scholastic Aptitude Test scores (SATs), and records of performance in extracurricular activities on and off the campus, we could explore relationships between findings from tests of students' academic abilities and performance and those of their serum chemical levels.

Obtaining permission

To obtain data such as the college students' laboratory test findings and records of academic progress, you must obtain permission from those in authority. This will require you to present a written description of your proposed research for their consideration.

The research proposal

The research proposal follows much the same format as a report for publication: (1) the *introduction* reviews the literature and provides an initial working hypothesis; (2) the *statement of the problem* states reasons for tackling the issue; (3) the *methods* section discusses the subjects, tests, and statistics to be used, and includes a description of the informed-consent procedure and form, if required; (4) the *results* section describes what you expect to find and how you plan to analyze and present results; and (5) the *discussion* explains what benefits may result from the research.

For the *Rape and Its Victims* study, it was necessary to obtain data from the public records and to conduct interviews with victims of sexual assault. Police reports of sexual assaults for the previous year were needed. Since this information is both personal and sensitive, it was necessary to establish credibility and rapport with local police officials. In the proposal to conduct the study, it was essential to assure the police of our professional integrity and of the strictly scientific nature of the research. In actually conducting the day-to-day gathering of data within the police setting, it was necessary to respect concerns of the police for confidentiality and to make certain that we did not interfere in the conduct of their duties. To ensure that data gathering could proceed smoothly when the time came, forms were prepared in advance. The forms were submitted to the police authorities in order to show the exact information that would be gleaned from their reports.

Collecting data in observed relation studies

In observed relation research you collect measurements of two or more variables and compare the data. Some examples of this stage of research are *naturalistic observations,* which were discussed previously, *surveys, epidemiological studies,* and *needs assessments.*

Survey research

Survey research is a form of field research where you go somewhere and observe what is happening there. You make your conditions of observation uniform and simplify your data analysis by using the same survey instrument. Surveys can also be used to learn about staff or patient attitudes or opinions, as will be shown later.

Epidemiological studies

These are concerned with incidence and prevalence of a disease or other condition in an area or community.

Incidence and prevalence. Studies that determine the incidence or prevalence of a disease in a community are always based on observed relations. *Incidence* refers to the actual occurrence of an event, such as the rate of occurrence of a specific disease among patients in a hospital. Incidence can indicate to what extent a population utilizes treatment resources. It is defined as the number of new cases of a particular condition within a population during a particular time period. Incidence rates are usually expressed per 100,000 population per year.

Prevalence is the degree to which a population is affected with a particular disease or condition at a given time: the percentage or rate of occurrence of the disease in the population as a whole. It is defined as the number of cases existing in a given population at any particular time. Prevalence indicates the population's need for services.

You can estimate prevalence by interviewing a random sample of a population in an area at a specified time and recording their responses on a structured interview or survey instrument. This method is expensive but potentially more accurate than the following procedures.

You can ask experts to give their estimates and analyze their replies. If you return the results of your analysis to the experts for them to think about, revise, refine, and return to you, the procedure is known as a *Delphi process*. Expert surveys are much less expensive than conducting a communitywide survey, because they require far fewer interviewers and subjects.

You can also obtain social indicator data from public records: rates of suicide, crime (especially infanticides and other homicides), death from psychosomatic disorders and cirrhosis, auto accidents (especially those associated with alcohol consumption), separation and divorce, juvenile delinquency, and the like. You can compare these rates to those of other communities and establish which communities have a significantly greater prevalence of various problems.

Studies with laboratory test equipment. Whenever you conduct an epidemiological study, you first must measure the reliability and validity of your questionnaires and other indicants.

To test the reliability of questionnaire responses in the epidemiologic survey, a large sample of the survey subjects underwent automated health testing. The subjects' reports on their survey questionnaires were compared with those they gave to the same questions at the health testing center. The test–retest intake data on demographic information ranged from 92.2% (for age) to 96.3% (for marital status). The agreement on selected disease symptoms was also good, ranging from 71% (for nervousness) to 96% (for loss of appetite); on treatment procedures, reliability ranged from 90.8% (for gynecological surgery) to 99.5% (for thyroidectomy) (R. E. Gordon, Warheit et al., 1975). Validity was measured by correlating symptoms reported on the survey instrument with actual findings of disease on biochemical and physiological tests.

Research with office patients. You can also examine your own and your colleagues' office records to check epidemiological trends about which you have made observed relation hypotheses. Of course you cannot express your findings in rates per 100,000 when you are presenting data from your own practice and those of your colleagues. You will generally use percentages.

Observed relation studies with private outpatients examined the hypothesis that periods of rapid community growth are associated with increased social stress and emotional disorder. Newcomers in fast-growing communities where retirees tend to settle, such as the counties of southernmost Florida, tend to need more psychiatric help than do natives of the area. Collier County grew by 68% in the period 1974 to 1984, and by 27% from 1980 to 1984. Disproportionately higher percentages of newcomers were among the psychiatric patients hospitalized in the county – 78% (as compared with 68% of the county's population as a whole) had lived in the county less than 10 years, and 53% (as compared to 27%) less than 4 years. The elderly, who were moving into the area at an especially high rate and providing between 23% and 30% of the region's population (the percentage varied by county), accounted for 50% of the patients in the area's private psychiatric hospital.

Depression, especially in the elderly, is often precipitated by loss. One of the main problems of socially mobile people is related to their loss of social supports – the comfort and help of family and old friends whom they left behind when they moved. Therefore, it causes no surprise that in Collier County's psychiatrists' offices the primary complaint of 67% of the patients is depression. By contrast, in Sarasota County, north of Collier County, where the population increased by only 14.3% in the 4-year period, only half as many – 33.5% – of the psychiatric office patients were depressed. These findings point to the need of socially mobile patients in rapidly growing communities for special preventive and treatment programs.

Research with community general hospital patients. The record room of the community general hospital provides an excellent resource for conducting epidemiological studies.

A study of psychosomatic problems in a rapidly growing suburb (R. E. Gordon & Gordon, 1959) obtained data on patient disease incidence from record rooms of three general hospitals located in widely separated communities that were growing at different rates. This study also investigated the hypothesis that rapid community growth is associated with increased emotional and psychosomatic disorder. Census reports gave the community growth-rate data. The communities were placed on an ordinal scale by growth rate. These rates were compared with percentages of patients with certain psychosomatic disorders who had received treatment in each hospital. Table 5.2 presents some of the data.

Note the relationship between growth rate and three psychosomatic diseases: coronary thrombosis, essential hypertension, and duodenal ulcer. The report also presented tables showing that in fast-growing Englewood, younger persons were more likely to develop psychosomatic disorders. Furthermore, the proportion of patients with psychosomatic diseases rose significantly in the Englewood hospital between the years 1950 and 1958, when the community underwent its most rapid growth. For example, there was a significant increase in coronary thrombosis and, among young women, in duodenal ulcer. These studies confirmed the hypothesis that rapid community growth is associated with increased psychosomatic disorder.

Table 5.2. *Observed relations between community growth rate and incidence of hospitalization for psychosomatic disorders (overall percentages of adult inpatients with the disorders)*

	Incidence of hospitalization		
Disease	Englewood	Kingston	Olean
Community growth rate	*7%*	*5%*	*4%*
Asthma	2.1	4.7	2.0
Coronary thrombosis	11.7	3.0	2.0
Essential hypertension	2.3	2.0	1.7
Hypertensive cardiovascular disease	12.0	3.2	5.0
Duodenal ulcer	9.6	7.1	2.8
Bronchopneumonia	7.3	5.3	5.0
Total no. of adult medical admissions	1,452	1,236	2,102

Studies with colleagues' and archival records. To cross-validate findings from one group of patients and remove any selection bias, you may review the records of patients of colleagues, the records of state mental hospitals serving several communities, and social indicator statistics obtained from state agencies and public archives.

We examined data on perinatal emotional disorder, suicide, infanticide, juvenile delinquency, separation, and divorce. Generally, these studies supported the basic observed relation hypothesis that rapid community growth is related to increased emotional disorder and other indicants of social distress (R. E. Gordon, Gordon & Gunther, 1961; R. E. Gordon, McWhorter, Singer & Gordon, 1960). For example, in the fast-growing southern part of the State of Florida the mean suicide rate in the early 1980s was 20.2 per 100,000 population, as compared with a mean of 14.9 in the northern part of the state. For the entire state, which is growing faster than the United States as a whole, the rate was 17, whereas for the nation the rate was 12.5.

Studies in court and administrative hearings. State officials, courts, agencies, and psychiatric hospitals are often interested in epidemiological data regarding communities' needs for psychiatric services. Sometimes states follow past utilization patterns in determining present psychiatric bed needs. This common method of estimating incidence and need makes the assumption that actual usage is related to need. However, patients may not seek help in a community's psychiatric facility for a number of reasons. For example, they may not perceive their need, they may not believe that the facilities can help them, or they may be referred to treatment centers outside the area.

Table 5.3. *Projections of psychiatric bed needs for an entire state illustrate the results of three methods of projecting needs*

Method of estimation	Projected need in year 1990
Utilization-based method	4,418
Delphi method	5,337
Epidemiologic survey method	5,813

Table 5.4. *Assessment of hospital bed needs in different areas of a state*

State district	Psychiatric hospital percentage occupancy	Rank by actual occupancy	Estimated bed need/ (surplus)	Rank by estimated need
5	54.6	9	(45)	4
4	58.9	8	2	6
2	62.2	7	(92)	3
1	62.7	6	58	9
3	67.2	5	(33)	5
10	72.1	4	22	7
7	72.3	3	(121)	2
6	74.6	2	48	8
11	82.0	1	(189)	1

Notes: This table provides data for the Spearman rank-order method of correlation (rho). Need has been estimated on the basis of past utilization. The list has been rank-ordered on the basis of increasing percentage of occupancy.

The rank-difference (rho) correlation between the two columns of rankings shown is .167. The table of significance of correlation coefficients in the Appendix shows that this correlation is not significantly different from zero (see chapter 5.A, "Computing Spearman's Rank Correlation").

Table 5.3 shows the results of three methods of predicting the need for inpatient psychiatric beds that were presented in a state administrative hearing. The utilization-based method estimated a private psychiatric bed need that was about 900 beds less than that projected by the Delphi method, and about 1,400 beds less than that obtained by the epidemiologic survey method.

State officials may assume that if there were a need for additional psychiatric services in a specific area, it would be reflected in higher occupancy rates in the area's local psychiatric facilities. The fallacy here is the same as that mentioned earlier: Patients in need may not enter a psychiatric hospital in an area.

Table 5.4 shows a comparison of actual occupancy rates in nine service areas in a state with need calculated by the utilization-based method. The areas have been ranked with those with the highest percentage of occupancy at the bottom of the table.

A *Spearman rank correlation coefficient (rho)* test of the observed relationship between the two columns of numbers shows that the relationship is not significantly different from zero. Thus the state's assumptions were without any basis in fact. These kinds of quantitative observed relation research data are very effective in impressing judges and juries.

Chapter 5.A shows you the simple procedure for computing the Spearman rank correlation coefficient, which is also called a *rank-order* or *rank-difference correlation coefficient.*

Spearman rank correlation coefficient (rho)

Spearman's rho is used when data are organized in ordinal rankings, as in Table 5.4. Ranking procedures work well when the number of variables is fairly small – fewer than 15 in number, as in Table 5.4. Kendall's tau is another statistic that measures the strength of a relationship between two sets of paired ranks. Later in this chapter we shall mention several more nonparametric statistical procedures you can use with ranked (ordinal) data. You can analyze data with these statistics on a microcomputer, as shown in chapter 5.A. But if you need to use a nonparametric statistical test other than Spearman's rho, seek the advice of a consultant for assistance as to which test to select and which computer program to use.

Needs assessments

In order to determine a patient's treatment needs, a hospital's or treatment unit's programmatic needs, or a community's psychiatric needs, you must generally perform assessments based on observed relation research. For example, in taking your depressed patient's psychosocial history you question her and her family carefully about possible losses she may have suffered. You know that high correlations have been observed between psychosocial losses and depression. Then when you design the program of a geriatric treatment unit you give special consideration to elderly patients' great likelihood to have undergone losses – of friends and loved ones, of physical health, of financial resources, and so on.

As shown before, you may use observed relation studies to determine psychiatric bed needs in a community. They also may help you to determine your patients' special treatment needs. Furthermore, they may help you monitor the effectiveness, costs, and efficiency of your treatment programs and office procedures and operations. If you use observed relation information to evaluate your policies and practices on a regular basis, you will be stimulated to think about how these might be changed and improved. Needs assessments lead to the planning and development of interventions. Later chapters will describe treatment programs designed to manage some patient problems identified in needs assessments.

Examples of needs assessments

Veteran psychiatric inpatients. A series of observed relation studies investigated the special characteristics and needs of veteran psychiatric patients as compared with those of nonveteran patients in a resort state. The studies showed that Veterans Administration psychiatric inpatient facilities tended to attract large numbers of transients who wandered from one part of the country to another. Forty-four percent of the veteran psychiatric inpatients studied had immigrated to the state within the past 10 years, as compared with 26% of nonveteran psychiatric patients and 19.5% of people in the state who did not require psychiatric hospitalization. The rootlessness, alienation, and lack of stable employment of these orbiting veteran patients created special problems for mental health facilities (R. E. Gordon, Lyons, Muniz & Most, 1973; Ogburn, Bellino, Williams & Gordon, 1969). (Chapter 3 noted that there was a bimodal age distribution among the veterans who participated in these studies, with about 59% of the patients being older men who had served in World War II or the Korean War, and the remaining 41% being younger veterans of the Vietnam War. An examination of the migratory tendencies of these two populations found that there were no significant differences.)

Observed relation studies that compared veteran psychiatric patients with nonveterans showed that the peripatetic veteran patient was characterized as follows: He was more likely (1) to be male; (2) not to work consistently in any one location; (3) not to cope with problems, but habitually to avoid and escape them by leaving, getting divorced, abandoning jobs, or entering a hospital; (4) to receive enough income from disability insurance, a pension, an inheritance, casual jobs, crime, or even investments to allow him to travel freely; (5) not to be married or, if married, to have marital and family problems; (6) to have been hospitalized previously in other states for psychiatric disorder; (7) to recover quickly after being hospitalized for illness, but not to cooperate in seeking outpatient aftercare; and (8) to be more likely than other veteran psychiatric patients to commit crimes (R. E. Gordon, Lyons et al., 1973; R. E. Gordon & Webb, 1975).

These findings contributed to a decision to unitize the psychiatric services of a veterans' psychiatric hospital on a geographic basis. The patients then received treatment from the same professionals both when hospitalized and in their aftercare.

Chronically ill mental patients. You can also assess patients' needs by obtaining the opinions of experts who are familiar with the patients, using the Delphi method mentioned previously.

This type of survey was conducted to determine the community placement needs of deinstitutionalized chronically ill mental patients, as shown in Table 5.5. Expe-

Table 5.5. *Needs assessment for state mental hospital geriatric patients' deinstitutionalization program (perceptions of experienced social service workers who work with elderly discharged mental patients)*

The best deinstitutionalization program imaginable	N	The worst deinstitutionalization program imaginable	N
1. Support systems for development of recreation, nutrition, health, peer support, etc.	37	1. Lack of patient prerelease training, preparation, or planning	23
2. Adequate residential placements with graduated levels of supervision and care	29	2. Lack of sufficient follow-up or aftercare	20
3. Comprehensive integration of services	29	3. Inadequate community outreach resources and support services	18
4. Appropriate placements	25	4. Lack of coordination and communication	15
5. Day-treatment programs	23	5. No program at all or fragmented health and social services	13
6. Good preplacement preparation and planning	22	6. "Dumping" clients anyplace that will take them	11
7. Adequate foster and boarding-home care	22	7. Little or no employee training and not enough qualified employees	10
8. Good follow-up and aftercare	21	8. Lack of consideration for patients' needs as individuals	9
9. Community awareness and involvement	17	9. Merely placing patients in foster or boarding homes	8
10. Qualified staff	17	10. Ignoring the elderly or isolating them	6
11. Prevention programs	16	11. Lack of case management and supervision	6
12. Proper funding	16	12. Not enough local programs and alternatives	5
13. Education and other activities built into residences	15	13. Lack of program and community residence assessment, evaluation, and supervision	4
14. Regular group therapy and skill building	15	14. Irresponsible or indiscriminate placement	4
15. Suitable locally available residences	11		
16. Effective referral system	11		
17. Disability determinations before release	11		
18. Regular service visits by case management	7		
19. Home care	6		
20. Transportation services	6		
21. Nursing home care	5		
22. Easy mobility to and from each level of care	3		

Note: One hundred and ten persons participated in the survey.
Source: Slater, Gordon, Patterson & Bowman, 1978.

Table 5.6. *Observed relationship between actual rapes and attempted rapes where assailant used a weapon (N = 55 interviewed subjects)*

Weapon	Rapes		Attempted rapes	
	No.	% of total	No.	% of total
Gun	4	12.5	4	17.4
Knife	12	37.5	5	21.7
Gun and knife	1	3.1	0	—
Other	2	6.2	0	—
Knife and other	1	3.1	0	—
Total cases where weapon was used	20	62.4	9	39.1
Total cases where no weapon was used	12	37.5	14	60.9
Total cases	32	100.0	23	100.0

z value for proportion of rapes with weapon vs. proportion of attempted rapes with weapon = 1.71. Proportions are not significantly different from each other.

rienced community agency workers whose jobs required that they come into daily contact with mental patients discharged from the state mental hospitals served as the experts for this study (Slater, Gordon, Patterson & Bowman, 1978).

These findings, along with other data, were used in planning both new modular psychoeducational treatment programs for chronic mental patients and a formal educational curriculum for state hospital employees in which they could obtain a junior college diploma. In order to evaluate the effectiveness of the state employees' training and education, they and their supervisors filled in survey forms after they had completed their program of studies. The supervisors compared the performance of the employees–students after training with their performance before training and with that of other supervisees. The students rated the overall education they received, the specific skills they learned, the individual courses they took, and their ability to apply what they had learned to their work (R. E. Gordon & Gordon, 1981: 184–9).

Victims of rape. The research on rape and its victims provides an example of another kind of needs assessment. It sought to determine what women need to know in order to prevent, avoid, or escape from sexual assault.

We interviewed women who had been sexually assaulted. Some of them had been raped, and some had been able to foil the attacker and escape before the rape was completed. Table 5.6 exhibits data from a total of 55 attacks, 32 of which were rapes and 23, attempted rapes. We were interested in whether or not there were differences in either situation or victim response associated with whether or not the attacker completed the rape (Hursch, 1977: 55).

In some attacks the offender carried a weapon. We compared the incidence of weapons in rapes and attempted rapes. Since the two groups did not have the same number of subjects, we used proportions to make them comparable.

Using the unit normal variate (z)

To do this comparison, we used the *unit normal variate* (*z*) and compared the proportion of rapes in which a weapon was used with the proportion of attempted rapes in which a weapon was used. The unit normal variate is used when it is necessary to compare scores that were recorded on two (or more) different scales. If, for example, we have a mean of 50 and a standard deviation of 10 recorded by one rater, and a mean of 210 and a standard deviation of 38 recorded by another rater, it would be difficult to compare the means of these two groups. This is where the *z* score, the unit normal variate, comes in handy. It will transform both sets of scores onto one "standard" scale. It will then be possible to compare them. The statistic *z* is based on the normal curve shown in Figure 2.2.

In the research on rape victims the question was "Is there a significant difference between the proportion of rapes where a weapon was used and the proportion of attempted rapes where a weapon was used?" If there were a significant difference, then we could infer that the absence of a weapon made a difference in whether or not a woman effectively resisted her attacker and prevented the rape.

For the data in Table 5.6, where 62.4% of the women who were raped faced an attacker with a weapon and only 39.1% of the women who resisted the rapist had to cope with a weapon, we obtained a *z* value of 1.71. (Chapter 5.A shows how to compute the *z* value.) Referring to the table of *z* values (see Appendix Table A.4), we found that the probability of obtaining this *z* value by chance was not high enough for us to consider the proportions significantly different. In other words, from these data alone we could not conclude that the presence of a weapon was a determining factor in whether or not a victim got raped. However, we still felt that this factor might play a role. We needed a larger sample of data. Therefore, we obtained police records of sexual assaults for an entire year and sorted those into completed rapes versus attempted rapes. Then we looked again at the presence or absence of a weapon. These data are shown in Table 5.7.

We again compared the proportion of rapes with a weapon to the proportion of attempted rapes with a weapon. The *z* value of 2.24 gave a probability of less than .02 that this result could occur by chance. Thus, by increasing the number of subjects (from 55 to 464) we were able to conclude that the proportions were significantly different. In terms of the variables, the study showed that an important difference in the situations where the victim got raped and those where she was successful in avoiding it was the presence of a weapon in the hands of her attacker. Our advice to women then was "Physical attack on a rapist is chancy if he has a weapon, but sometimes worth the risk if he does not" (Hursch, 1977: 161).

Students' serum chemicals, grades, and other measures. Several studies of college students' needs examined relationships between their serum chemicals, their scholastic aptitudes and grades, and their extracurricular activities. Table 5.8 presents product-moment correlation coefficients (*r*) between students' Scholastic Aptitude Test (SAT) scores, grade-point averages (GPAs), serum uric acid (SUA) levels, and serum cholesterol (CHOL) levels. (Chapter 5.A discusses the product-

Table 5.7. *Observed relationship between actual rapes and attempted rapes where assailant used a weapon (N = 464 reported assaults)*

	Rapes		Attempted rapes	
Weapon	No.	% of total	No.	% of total
Gun	63	21.0	26	15.8
Knife	92	30.7	43	26.2
Gun and knife	3	1.0	1	0.6
Gun and other	0	0	1	0.6
Knife and other	2	0.7	0	0
Other	17	5.7	8	4.9
Total cases where weapon was used	177	59.0	79	48.2
Total cases where no weapon was used	123	41.0	85	51.8

z value for proportion of rapes with weapon vs. proportion of attempted rapes with weapon = 2.24; $p < .02$. Proportions are significantly different from each other.

Table 5.8. *Correlational data on college students' academic and serum chemical variables (illustrates the use of Pearson's product-moment correlation)*

	SAT	GPA	SUA	
Females: GPA	.29**	.27**		$N = 70$
SUA	.09			
	CHOL	−.10	.18*	.083
Males: GPA	.30**			
SUA	.11	.22**		$N = 75$
CHOL	.08	.05	−.02	

Note: SAT = Scholastic Aptitude Test; GPA = grade-point average; SUA = serum uric acid; CHOL = cholesterol.
*Significant at the .05 level. ** Significant at the .01 level.

moment correlation coefficient, r.) Table 5.8 shows that for both male and female students SUA and SAT were slightly, but significantly (r ranged from .22 to .30; $p < .01$), correlated with GPA. Cholesterol was significantly ($p < .05$) correlated with female students' GPAs, but not with male students' GPAs (Lindeman et al., 1969).

In this example, serum chemical (uric acid and cholesterol) levels, SAT scores, and GPAs were all assessed in the form of continuous, interval scale variables.

Therefore, parametric statistics (means, standard deviations, *t* tests, and product-moment correlations – *r*) apply. Chapter 5.A describes how these indexes were used to compute product-moment correlations.

Pearson's product-moment correlation coefficient (r)

Pearson's product-moment correlation coefficient is used in about 7% of articles in the major psychiatric journals (Hokanson et al., 1986). Chapter 5.A shows how to compute it from the raw data.

There are two other correlation coefficients that you will run across – the *point biserial coefficient of correlation* and the *tetrachoric correlation*. The first is used when one variable is continuous and the other is dichotomous or in a twofold classification, such as when items are scored 1 if correct and 0 if incorrect. Point biserial is useful in item analysis. Tetrachoric correlation, which is a modified form of product-moment correlation, is used when both variables are assumed to be continuous, but the only values you have on each are dichotomous. You then have a two-by-two table. You can obtain software programs for the microcomputer to calculate these and other correlation coefficients, as shown in Chapter 5.A.

Multivariate statistics and examples

The following studies utilized highly technical multivariate statistics and correlational data involving large numbers of variables. These multivariate techniques handle many variables in a single analysis. We present these more complicated statistics for handling complexity – discriminant analysis, factor analysis, analysis of variance, and multiple regression analysis – to acquaint you with their names and purposes so that you will recognize and understand what they do when you run across them in your reading. They are all parametric statistical procedures that require interval or ratio scale data. These last are frequently unavailable in psychiatric research. Watch out when they are used by persons whose expertise is questionable.

If you decide to tackle complicated multivariate research, you can use microcomputers to perform the analyses of the data. However, before you attempt any of the following procedures we recommend that you obtain help from a consultant in statistics or experimental design.

Discriminant function analysis. Discriminant function analysis can be used to classify patients/subjects into groups, such as diagnostic categories. Suppose you have obtained test scores on a large sample of psychiatric patients, some of whom have been given *DSM-III* diagnoses. You can use discriminant function analysis to determine the best way to combine scores on the various tests in order to identify which patients in the group at large should be assigned to each diagnostic subgroup.

Discriminant analysis of admissions to a Veterans Administration hospital. A study of the admission process at a Veterans Administration hospital used discriminant analysis. Among veterans who applied for admission to the hospital, 241 went through an automated multiphasic health testing center (R. E. Gordon, 1971). The veterans underwent a battery of tests and procedures. The discriminant analysis determined which psychiatric test scores, physiological tests, and chemical tests (all are continuous, interval scale variables) were related to where the patient was referred – to the medical, the surgical, or the psychiatric service. It also determined what admission decision was made – to admit or not to admit the patient to the hospital (nominal scale criterion). The best discriminating combination was made up of items from the psychiatric battery (R. E. Gordon, Bielen & Watts, 1973; R. E. Gordon, Holzer, et al., 1973).

Factor analysis. By analyzing product-moment correlation coefficients among a large set of variables, factor analysis finds which variables are close enough to each other to suggest that they can be combined into a single factor or class. Both factor analysis and discriminant analysis appear only rarely in the psychiatric literature (Hokanson et al., 1986).

Factor analyses with data from the maternity questionnaire (see chapter 4) showed that the questionnaire measures two main factors. The first factor is related to personal insecurity arising out of the new mother's personal background stresses; the second is associated with conflict in her new maternal role related to her lack of adequate social support (Gartner & Riessman, 1982; R. E. Gordon, Kapostins & Gordon, 1965). These early findings of the importance of aggravating stresses and environmental supports in patients' lives have been cited frequently in the medical and psychological literature.

Multiple regression analysis. When you have more than two interval or ratio-scaled variables, you can perform a multiple regression analysis and obtain a multiple correlation coefficient (R). Multiple regression analysis allows you to study the relationship between a set of independent variables and a dependent variable while taking into account the interrelationships (or intercorrelations) among the independent variables. The combination can then be used to predict the effect of each on the dependent variable. Regression analysis appears in about 3% of the psychiatric literature (Hokanson et al., 1986).

For example, scores on the maternity questionnaire were obtained from a group of expectant mothers in the first trimester of pregnancy. Subsequently, during their pregnancies and in the six months postpartum, they counted their numbers of crying spells. After delivery, their emotional reactions were measured on a standardized psychosocial instrument – the Leighton scale (Leighton, 1963). In the second and third antenatal trimesters, the women's estriol levels were also assessed. The hypothesis was that maternity questionnaire scores would predict numbers of prenatal crying spells and estriol levels, and that the combination of questionnaire scores, crying-spell counts, and hormonal levels would predict postnatal emotional state. Table 5.9 presents the findings of the study (R. E. Gordon, Gordon, Gordon-Hardy, Hursch & Reed, 1986). The significance levels of the correlations in Table 5.9 are obtained from Appendix Table A.3.

The multiple correlation coefficient (R) was .94 between the three predictor variables and the criterion variable: postpartum emotional reaction. The combination of maternity questionnaire scores early in pregnancy, which measured the aggravating stress and environmental supports in their lives, and numbers of crying spells and hormonal levels, which assessed their subsequent biomedical status, was highly predictive of postpartum emotional state.

In other multiple regression analyses, data on the five axes of *DSM-III*, the strain ratio (the ratio of Axis IV to Axis V), severity of illness, and demographic information (age and sex) were combined in a regression equation. The multiple correlation coefficient (R) of this multiaxial combination with length of stay (LOS) in a psychiatric hospital ranged between .64 and .78, and R^2 ranged between .41 and .62. In other words, this combination predicted between 41% and 62% of the variability in LOS (R. E. Gordon, Vijay et al., 1985).

The new edition of the *Diagnostic and Statistical Manual of Mental Disorders,* third edition, *DSM-III-R* (American Psychiatric Association, 1987), calls for including a rating of current severity of the disorder. Further research is needed with *DSM-III-R* to check the above findings. However, the findings suggest that "a multiaxial diagnostic approach that assesses level of functioning, psychosocial stressors, and presence of personality disorders appears to have promise in predicting length of stay" (Caton & Gralnick, 1987). If new studies replicate the finding above, they may indicate that a basic law applies in psychiatry as in other medical specialties: *Diagnosis determines treatment need.*

You can obtain useful findings with analysis of variance, regression analysis, and other multivariate procedures that you can conduct in your office. You need only test your patients, consult a statistician, and use a microcomputer.

Some more nonparametric tests and examples

There is a wide variety of nonparametric tests besides those described previously that you can use when you do not have interval or ratio-scaled

Table 5.9. *Product-moment correlations among antenatal and postnatal measures of stress, hormones, crying, and emotional reaction*

| Measure | N | Antenatal trimesters | | | Postnatal trimesters | | | |
| | | First | Third | | First | | Second | |
		ASymp 1 16	Estr 3 13	ACry 3 16	PSymp 1 40	PCry 1 16	PSymp 2 13	PCry 2 16
First antenatal trimester								
Stress Q	40				.49****			
Asymp 1	16	.69****	−.55**	.61**[u125]*	.58***	.56***	.64***	.53**
Second antenatal trimester								
Estr 2	16		.65***					
ACry 2	16		−.57**	.53**				
Third antenatal trimester								
Estr 3	13			−.67***	.67****		−.47*	
ACry 3	16					.72*****		.76*****

Abbreviations

Stress Q = Antenatal stress questionnaire
ASymp 1 = Antenatal symptom scale
Estr 2 = Estriol level, second antenatal trimester
ACry 2 = Number of crying spells, second antenatal trimester
Estr 3 = Estriol level, third antenatal trimester
ACry 3 = Number of crying spells, third antenatal trimester

PSymp 1 = Symptom scale score, first postnatal trimester
PSymp 2 = Symptom scale score, second postnatal trimester
PCry 2 = Number of crying spells, second postnatal trimester
Only correlations of .47 or better are shown. Significance: * = .10.
** = .05. *** = 0.25. **** = .01. ***** = .001.

Table 5.10. *Using the Wilcoxon matched-pairs signed-ranks test to compare sleep stages of prepartum, postpartum, and nonpregnant women (mean sleep time in minutes)*

Stage	Prepartum (Nights 2 & 3)	Postpartum (Nights 2 & 3)	Control (2½ or 4 mo.)	Nonpregnant
0	34 · 80 c** np**	38 · 91 c** np**	9 · 50 np*	3 · 33
1	30 · 19	23 · 29	20 · 25	26 · 91
1-REM	77 · 65 np**	74 · 37 np*	82 · 00	99 · 08
2	225 · 73 c**	165 · 37 np*	176 · 92 np*	224 · 66
3	19 · 73	22 · 45	21 · 08	26 · 50
4	37 · 11 c** np**	47 · 66 c**	75 · 08	67 · 91
Total	425 · 21	372 · 05	384 · 83	448 · 39

c** = significantly different from control ($p < .01$).

np** = significantly different from nonpregnant ($p < .01$).

c* = significantly different from control ($p < .05$).

np* = significantly different from nonpregnant ($p < .05$).

data in your research. The examples that follow show the use of some of them.

Table 5.10 shows the mean time spent in each of the six EEG sleep stages by prepartum, postpartum, control, and nonpregnant women (Karacan, Williams, Hursch, McCaulley & Heine, 1969). For comparing the prepartum and postpartum groups with the control group, the nonparametric *Wilcoxon matched-pairs signed-ranks test* was used, since the same women were tested during their prepartum, postpartum, and control (one week after reestablishment of the menses) periods. The Wilcoxon test is a nonparametric statistical test that gives weight to both direction and magnitude of the differences between pairs. This test was used because the same subjects were involved; therefore the samples are *related.*

The *Mann–Whitney U test* was used for comparing the pregnant women's sleep patterns with those of the nonpregnant women, since the two groups consisted of two different sets of subjects and are therefore *independent* samples. This test is a powerful nonparametric test that you can use when your data cannot satisfy the assumptions for a *t* test.

Table 5.11 compares sleep patterns of insomniacs with those of controls. Some of the comparisons in Table 5.11 (Karacan, Williams, Salis & Hursch, 1971) were made by means of the parametric *t* test, but note that for one variable, latency of

Table 5.11. *Using the sign test for comparing sleep patterns of insomniacs and controls*

| | Night 1 | | | | Later nights | | | |
| | Insomniacs | | Controls | | Insomniacs | | Controls | |
Variable	Mean	SD	Mean	SD	Mean	SD	Mean	SD
Sleep latency	56.80	51.84**	8.30	7.24	37.80	26.83**	10.65	5.68
Total sleep time	281.60	134.29*	386.20	23.89	340.67	87.65	391.25	32.41
Sleep efficiency	0.66	0.28**	0.94	0.04	0.81	0.14*	0.93	0.07
Latency of arising	34.10	38.24*	2.20	4.73	14.37	15.99*	2.55	4.85
% slow-wave sleep	4.33	6.94*	11.44	10.84	8.59	11.87	12.68	7.80
Latency of slow-wave sleep[a,b]	58.00	93.57	36.44	26.21	60.04	34.21*	28.56	16.88
% stage 0	16.21	18.13*	3.12	2.94	6.65	6.44	4.50	5.68

[a] $N = 4$ for insomniacs, Night 1; $N = 9$ for controls, Night 1, and for insomniacs and controls, later nights.
[b] Sign test for Night 1 comparison.
*Significantly different ($p < .05$, one-tailed) from controls.
**Significantly different ($p < .01$, one-tailed) from controls.

slow-wave sleep, the comparison between insomniacs and controls for Night 1 was made by means of the nonparametric *sign test*. This was owing to the fact that only four of the insomniacs had any slow-wave sleep on Night 1. Therefore it was impossible to use the *t* test, because it is not reliable for a group that small. It was possible to use the sign test here. However, it resulted in no significant difference between the group scores. The sign test uses information about the direction but not the magnitude of the differences within pairs.

Other nonparametric statistical tests

The *Fisher exact probability test* is a valuable nonparametric test for analyzing discrete nominal or ordinal data when the size of the two independent samples is small. You can use it with independent samples measured on nominal scales. The *Kolmogorov–Smirnov one-sample test* is concerned with the goodness of fit between the distribution of a set of values (observed scores) and some theoretical distribution. The *Kolmogorov–Smirnov two-sample test* is a test of whether or not two independent samples are drawn from the same underlying population; that is, whether or not the variable you are measuring has the same type of distribution for the two groups. For example, a variable like aggression (defined on a specified scale), plotted against intelligence level, may be normally distributed in one group but may be skewed toward the lower end in the other group. Or it may have a higher mean value in one group than the other, or it may be more variable (have a larger standard deviation) in one group than the other. The Kolmogorov–Smirnov two-sample test will pick up any of these differences in distribution.

The *median test* determines whether two independent groups possibly of different sizes have been drawn from populations with the same medians. These tests are described in detail in Siegel (1957).

Statistical software and a microcomputer can help you perform these nonparametric statistical tests. However, you should call in a consultant for assistance about which test to select and which computer program to use.

Writing up results

In 1959 newspapers across the nation displayed headlines like "Crabgrass, Taxes and Tension Breeding Ailments in Suburbs." They were reporting on the lead article in the current issue of the *Journal of the American Medical Association,* the report "Psychosomatic Problems of a Rapidly Growing Suburb" (R. E. Gordon & Gordon, 1959). Unfortunately, the headline was not accurate. In writing up and reporting findings from observed relation research, you cannot draw causal conclusions when they are based only on correlations between two variables. You cannot state that suburban life causes ulcers or other illnesses. The study only showed that there was a relationship between community growth and emotional distress. Perhaps vulnerable people move more than others. Or stresses due to changing homes and jobs or to loss of support from family and friends may contribute to emotional and psychosomatic problems. The community itself may make it hard on newcomers. Or other factors may explain the findings better.

You must be very careful when you find an abnormal image on patient brain scans, for example, to resist inferring that it caused the associated psychiatric disease. First you must show that other factors did not result in both the defective anatomical development and the disease. To do this you must conduct well-controlled causal relation research.

Summary

This chapter has discussed observed relation or correlational research, which is commonly found in psychiatric and other medical journals. It has also presented examples of multivariate and some complicated nonparametric statistics. You can conduct observed relation studies in office practice with little or no cost. However, research based on simple correlation alone cannot imply causality or suggest easy solutions to problems.

The chapter has continued the exploration of the concepts of aggravating stress and functional level, showing that they are correlated with amount of social mobility in a community. Many observed relation studies assess and monitor patients' treatment needs. Epidemiological surveys are conducted in observed relation research. Assessments of hospitals' and communities' needs are also based on correlational studies. They may suggest ideas for subsequent controlled experiments, including new approaches to treatment.

Most observed relation studies use simple nonparametric and parametric statistics to provide the relationships between data when only two variables are present. Multivariate statistics may be used when you are examining the effects of more than two variables. You should employ the services of a consultant when you use multivariate or complicated nonparametric statistics.

5.A. More simple statistics

More nonparametric statistics

Computing Spearman's rank correlation (rho)

This computation is easy. Let us consider the ranks of the actual occupancy in psychiatric hospitals versus the estimated need by the state formula described in Table 5.4. Table 5.A.1 provides the calculations for the data in that table.

Table 5.A.2 shows the output from the microcomputer analysis of the same data.

Table 8.6 provides another example of the use of Spearman's rank correlation (rho) that, in this case, is statistically significant. The calculations for the correlation between the strain ratio (SR) and the amount of treatment the patients required are shown in Table 5.A.3.

More parametric statistics

Computing the unit normal variate (z)

The unit normal variate (z) was used to compute the significance of differences between proportions in Tables 5.7 and 5.8. Table 5.A.4 shows how to perform the calculations in Table 5.7.

Computing Pearson's product-moment coefficient of correlation

The formula for calculating Pearson's product-moment correlation coefficient (r) is as follows:

$$r = [N\Sigma(xy) - (\Sigma x)(\Sigma y)] / \sqrt{[N\Sigma x^2 - (x)^2][N\Sigma y^2 - (y)^2]}$$

116

Table 5.A.1. *The calculation of a Spearman rank correlation coefficient (rho) where the rho is not significant*

Rank by actual occupancy	Rank by estimated need	Difference	
		(D)	D^2
9	4	5	25
8	6	2	4
7	3	4	16
6	9	3	9
5	5	0	0
4	7	3	9
3	2	1	1
2	8	6	36
1	1	0	0
Sum of the squares (ΣD^2)			100

First subtract each pair and put the difference in the third column above, as shown. Sum the difference-squared (D^2) column, obtaining the number 100. Put it, the number of subjects (N), and their square (N^2) in the following formula:

$$\text{rho} = 1 - \frac{6\Sigma D^2}{N(N^2 - 1)}$$

Filling in the formula:

$$\text{rho} = 1 - \frac{6 \times 100}{9(81 - 1)} = 1 - (600/720) = .167$$

Referring to Appendix Table A.6, we find that for an N of 9 we need a rho of .600 to be significant at the .05 level and of .783 to reach the .01 level. Thus the rho above of .167 is not significant.

Table 5.A.2. *A microcomputer analysis of the data in Table 5.A.1*

Spearman Corr. Coef.   X : Percentage Occupancy   Y : Estimated Bed Need

N	9
ΣD^2	100
Rho	.167
Z	.471

Table 5.A.3. *The calculation of a Spearman rank correlation coefficient (rho) where the rho is significant*

Strain ratio	0.73	0.85	0.97[a]	0.90	0.97[a]	1.03	1.25
Rank of strain ratio	1	2	4.5[a]	3	4.5[a]	6	7
Rank of amount of treatment	1	2	3	4	5	6	7
Difference (D)	0	0	1.5	-1	-0.5	0	0
D^2	0	0	2.25	1	0.25	0	0 = 3.5

Sum $D^2 = 3.5$

$$\text{rho} = 1 - \frac{6\Sigma D^2}{N(N^2 - 1)} = 1 - \frac{6 \times 3.5}{7 \times 48} = 1 - .0625 = .94$$

Referring again to Appendix Table A.6, we now see that for an N of 7, a rho of .94 is significant beyond the .01 level.

[a]When there are two or more tied scores, each receives the average of the ranks that would have been assigned if no ties had occurred. The fourth- and fifth-ranked SR values were both .97. We sum 4 and 5 and divide by 2, getting 4.5 as the number to use.

Table 5.A.4. *The calculation of the unit normal variate (z)*

	Rapes		Attempted rapes	
	No.	% of total	No.	% of total
Weapon used	20	62.4	9	39.1
No weapon used	12	37.5	14	60.9
Total cases	32	100.0	23	100.0

The formula for z is:

$$z = (p_1 - p_2)/\sqrt{pqN/N_1N_2}$$

where p_1 is the first proportion, p_2 the second proportion, $p = (N_1p_1 + N_2p_2)/(N_1 + N_2)$, $q = (1 - p)$, and $N = N_1 + N_2$.
Putting in the numbers,

$$N_1p_1 = 32 \times .624; \; N_2p_2 = 23 \times .391; \text{ and } N_1 + N_2 = 55$$

Therefore, $p = (32 \times .624 + 23 \times .391)/55 = (19.97 + 8.99)/55 = 28.96/55 = .527$.
And $q = 1 - p = .473$.
Also, $p_1 - p_2 = .624 - .391 = .233$.
Filling in these numbers in the formula for z:

$$z = (.624 - .391)/\sqrt{(.527)(.473)(55)/(32)(23)} = .233/.136 = 1.71$$

The z value for proportion of rapes with weapon versus proportion of attempted rapes with weapon = 1.71. Reference to Appendix Table A.4 reveals that the proportions are significantly different from each other.

Table 5.A.5. *The calculation of Pearson's product-moment correlation coefficient when deviations are taken from two distributions*

Football player	Spring uric acid level	Fall uric acid level	x_s	y_f	x^2	y^2	xy
A	6	7	1	0	1	0	0
B	4	6	-1	-1	1	1	1
C	3	5	-2	-2	4	4	4
D	7	9	2	2	4	4	4
E	5	8	0	1	0	1	0
F	7	6	2	-1	4	1	-2
G	3	4	-2	-3	4	9	6
H	6	9	1	2	1	4	2
I	4	7	-1	0	1	0	0
J	5	9	0	2	0	4	0
Total	50	70	0	0	20	28	15
Mean$_s$ = 5 Mean$_f$ = 7			(x)	(x)	(x^2)	(y^2)	(xy)

$$r = [N\Sigma(xy) - (\Sigma x)(\Sigma y)]/\sqrt{[N\Sigma x^2 - (x)^2][N\Sigma y^2 - (y)^2]}$$

where x_s and y_f are deviations from the spring and fall means, Mean$_s$ and Mean$_f$, respectively. Putting in the numbers:

$$r = (10)(15) - (0)(0)/\sqrt{(10)(0 - 20)(10)(0 - 28)} =$$

$$r = (150)/\sqrt{(-200)(-280)} = 150/236.64 = .634$$

Referring now to Appendix Table A.3, we see that for 10 subjects a correlation of .634 is significant beyond the .05 level.

Table 5.A.6. *A microcomputer analysis of the data in Table 5.A.5*

Corr. Coeff. X : Spring Uric Acid Level	Y : Fall Uric Acid Level		
Count:	**Covariance:**	**Correlation:**	**R-squared:**
10	1.667	.634	.402

In Table 5.A.5, x and y are deviations from the means of the two groups. This table contains 10 football players' spring and fall serum uric acid levels. (Data have been rounded to whole numbers for ease of computation in the illustration.)

Table 5.A.6 shows the microcomputer analysis of the same data.

Suggestions for further reading

1. Mark Finkelstein, *Statistics at Your Fingertips*. Belmont, CA: Wadsworth, 1985. An excellent self-teaching text, written for use with hand calculators of several different types. Step-by-step procedures and illustrations. Very readable. Parametric and nonparametric statistics.

2. Paul Karoly (ed.), *Measurement Strategies in Health Psychology*. New York: Wiley, 1985. Collected papers of leading researchers on skillful methods of getting at subtle variables.

3. Michael J. Lambert, Edwin R. Christensen & Steven S. DeJulio (eds.), *The Assessment of Psychotherapy Outcome*. New York: Wiley, 1983. A collection of papers by experts describing different approaches to the evaluation of treatment programs.

4. David W. Martin, *Doing Psychology Experiments,* 2d ed. Monterey, CA: Brooks/Cole, 1985. A very readable, humorously written book on serious research. Starts with such basics as how to plan an experiment, choosing variables, and writing reports, and proceeds through more complicated statistical concepts. Parametric and nonparametric statistics.

5. Richard P. Runyon, *Fundamentals of Statistics in the Biological, Medical, and Health Sciences*. Boston: Duxbury, 1985. A well-written, clearly laid-out text with many applications to branches and specialties within the subject fields. Comprehensive. Starts with the basics and proceeds with much explanatory material through all of the commonly used parametric and nonparametric statistics.

6. Sidney Siegel, *Nonparametric Statistics for the Behavioral Sciences*. New York: McGraw-Hill, 1957. Despite the age of this text, it is still widely used by researchers who work with human beings. It is undoubtedly the most complete practical text available on nonparametrics. Its charts and clear presentation make it easy to locate the right test for your purposes. Written before hand calculators and personal computers were popular, it stresses the least arduous method of computing each statistic.

6. Observed causal research

It is much harder to conduct well-controlled experimental research with psychiatric patients than with laboratory animals or biological specimens. In an experiment you perform some research procedure on one (or more) variable(s) and measure the resulting changes (if any) in another variable. You do this because your research hypothesis states that changes in the target (or dependent) variable are due to the changes that your treatment imposes on the existing (or independent) variable. The *independent variable* is the condition manipulated or selected by the experimenter to determine its effect on behavior. The *dependent variable* is a measure of the behavior of the patient/subject that reflects the effects of the independent variable (McBurney, 1983).

You hold constant or control any extraneous variables. In desk-top laboratory studies you encounter little difficulty in assigning specimens to either control or experimental groups, but in human research this conceptually simple procedure runs into many barriers. Not only psychiatric studies, but those in other service-delivery settings that, for example, test the benefits of rehabilitation programs in prisons, bilingual education in schools, even new mathematics programs in elementary school, run into obstacles in the use of human control groups.

You generally must perform clinical research that attempts to benefit the patient. Risky or painful experimental studies of the effects of stress or brain injury, for example, can usually be done only on experimental animals.

It is very difficult to conduct research into the benefits of new therapies without administrative control over the patient population. Investigators who try to impose a controlled research study upon someone else's treatment unit frequently meet with frustration. Thus in many clinical situations you will find that you are introducing a new program with incomplete controls. You often must content yourself, at least in preliminary

121

studies, with evaluating the benefits of a program with partially controlled *observed causal research* methods, rather than in fully controlled *causal relation research,* which is described in the next chapter.

Definition

A research has reached the *observed causal* stage if it fulfills the following criteria:

1. There are (at least) two measured variables
2. There are two or more values of a treatment variable, which may or may not be under the control of the experimenter
3. There are one or more dependent variables. There must be two (or more) measures of each dependent variable, corresponding to two (or more) values of the treatment variable

In a true causal relation experiment you have complete control over the experiment and can randomly assign subjects/patients to the various conditions. You can manipulate the variables at will. In an observed causal or quasi-experiment you lack this degree of control; you must generally select subjects for the different conditions from previously existing groups after they have already been formed. You can only observe the subjects.

You can sometimes turn treatment settings into clinical research laboratories if you are in charge of your own ward in a hospital, clinic, or individual patient practice. You can consider each clinical treatment of a patient to be part of a research experiment with a group of patients/subjects that compares the patients' pretreatment conditions with those after discharge. Sometimes you may be able to control most of the relevant variables in working with a single patient/subject. In that case, the main reservations that apply have to do with extrapolating the results of this case to other cases. The reason for using more subjects is to nullify the effect of individual differences. You have no way of knowing whether any one subject is above or below average or right on the mean in his response to your experimental treatment or procedure.

In most medical treatment studies, having 80% of the patients respond positively to the treatment is an exciting and positive result. If you use only one subject and do not get a positive response, you do not know whether your treatment is beneficial and this patient is one of the 20% who do not respond to it or if your treatment has no effect. Similarly, if you use one subject and get a positive response, you may have a treatment to which only 10% of your patients will respond positively and this happens to be one of those who do. However, you can accumulate patients on whom you try the treatment one by one and build up a treatment group that way. Then the individual differences among patients will cancel each other out, and you will be getting results based on your treatment rather than on their individual differences.

Waiting-list controls

When you can control admissions to a clinic or other treatment setting where patients must wait to be treated, you can sometimes obtain controls for evaluating a new treatment by randomly assigning patients either to the treatment group(s) or to the waiting list. Although there may be some ethical objections to your assigning patients to a waiting list, these are minimized when all patients are eventually treated.

Using patients as their own controls

In this procedure you test the patients before the treatment is applied and again after it is applied. In this way, you actually have only one group of subjects, but you have two sets of measures of the dependent variable – one before treatment and one after. In this design, since the subjects are their own controls, the experimental group is perfectly matched with the control group on all variables. This kind of research design is possible in drug studies, but only if you allow enough time for the effects of one drug to wear off before you give another to the same patients.

It is also commonly used in before-and-after experiments, where you can measure a trait or characteristic accurately before a treatment is applied and again afterward. For example, the effectiveness of a weight-loss program could be tested using this method. Several measures of obesity can be taken before the subjects start on the program. Then measures could again be taken at three-month intervals after treatment begins. In this way, all subjects' indexes are compared with their own previous data. Measures are obtained for comparison just as though the first measures (before starting the program) were the control measures and the three-month measurements were the experimental ones. The significance of the differences can then be computed for the group.

There are many other before-and-after situations where this method can be applied. It is especially useful because it results in the most closely matched control group possible.

There are some pitfalls associated with using patients as their own controls. For example, if you wish to test the effects of a new medication upon the short-term memory of aged patients using them as their own controls, you may give a memory test to these subjects. Then you administer the special new medication before giving them the memory test at a later session. At this point, you must use a different form of the test to avoid a "practice effect." If you do not, there may be some carryover from the first session.

Another problem is that the control and experimental phases of the experiment take place at different periods in time. Events in the lives of the patients outside the control of the experimenter might affect their responses.

Program evaluation

Whenever you administer a new drug or other therapy (independent variable) to a group of patients, you are potentially doing an experiment if you also carefully measure the changes in the patients' behavior (dependent variable). Clinically, program evaluations determine whether a new treatment is producing better results with a group of patients than were achieved before the treatment became available. However, in clinical practice you may need to evaluate the effectiveness of a new program of therapy without being able to design an experiment where you can control nonexperimental variables. If you conduct such a partially controlled observed causal or quasi-experimental study, you must recognize that you cannot place the same amount of confidence in the findings about the new treatment's effects as you can when you exercise the kind of control described in the chapter on causal relation research. The sections that follow describe three quasi-experimental program evaluations.

Examples of observed causal research

All three of the observed causal research investigations described below were undertaken after observed relation research helped assess the needs of each population for whom the treatment program was designed. Each treatment program attempted to improve the patients' functioning. The Axis V scale was not yet available to measure this dependent variable, so other measures were used. The *combined treatment of psychiatric outpatients* (R. E. Gordon, 1959; R. E. Gordon, Gordon & Gunther, 1961) was designed to meet the needs of private patients who lived in rapidly growing communities. The *geographic unitization of a veterans' hospital psychiatric program* was organized to help the "orbiting" veteran patient. The *modular psychoeducational treatment of chronic mental patients* was developed to prepare state hospital geriatric inpatients for living in the community outside the hospital (R. E. Gordon & Gordon, 1981).

The studies that follow were conducted temporally in the sequence shown: The combined treatment studies were performed in the 1950s and early 1960s, when psychotropic medications were first becoming available. It examined the effectiveness of eclectic treatment that combined dynamic, pharmacological, behavioral, and social therapies in the clinical care of psychiatric patients.

The geographic unitization research took place in the late 1960s and early 1970s. It evaluated the usefulness of continuity of care in providing veteran patients with social support and continued psychiatric treatment after they left the hospital, treatment approaches that were also explored in the combined treatment work. It also employed a standardized rating scale, since these were beginning to be developed.

The modular psychoeducational investigations were conducted in the late 1970s. They examined other features of the combined treatment studies – the use of formal psychoeducational classes with modular course materials to help patients and their families learn a variety of coping skills. It utilized a number of standardized rating scales and other psychosocial instruments to assess patients' needs and progress in treatment. Thus, the modular psychoeducational research served to follow up on the social behavioral aspects of the earlier combined treatment research.

Moreover, it offered a considerable improvement in its scientific methodology over traditional psychotherapy. In traditional psychotherapy, (1) patients generally work out their own solutions, discussing what comes to mind each session, with no order of priority. (2) Periodically, therapists may provide them with an insight, suggest a way of behaving, or instruct them, but not according to any preplanned, methodical system. (3) Important problems in the patient's behavior and functioning may be ignored unless the patient brings them up. (4) There is no built-in assessment of the extent of the problem nor the progress the patient has made in overcoming it, although the therapist can require periodic independent testing. (5) Data cannot routinely be pooled and compared, since there is no routine systematic testing of patients' progress.

In contrast, each module in psychoeducational treatment contains, in addition to other elements: (1) a clearly defined psychoeducational goal,

(2) a statement of behavioral objectives, (3) a standardized pretest that is given before the main content of the course, (4) the procedures by which the patient can achieve each behavioral objective, (5) standardized assessments that measure the patient's improving proficiency during treatment; and (6) a standardized posttest that follows completion of the main content. Furthermore, modular data from groups of patients can be pooled, compared, and contrasted, since each module uses the same tests to assess patients.

Hypotheses for combined treatment study with private psychiatric outpatients

Studies of psychiatric outpatients, inpatients, and psychosomatic patients were conducted with office private patients in the 1950s. These studies assessed suburban patients' special characteristics and needs. They led to hypotheses that many patients were unskilled in coping with the stress of moving into and living in new suburban communities, and that many were receiving inadequate support from family, friends, and community. Positive findings from studies of maternity psychiatric patients and of women in antenatal classes and their husbands provided information about the coping and social support needs of patients and their families.

Traditionally, there had been two main kinds of psychiatric treatments prior to these studies: (1) Psychodynamically oriented psychotherapy was usually provided to outpatients. It usually excluded the family of adult patients. (2) Shock therapies – insulin, electroconvulsive, and sometimes metrazol – mostly required inpatient care. In the new treatment approach we hypothesized that patients would benefit from a combination of psychotropic medications, as needed; behavioral training that included extinction of unrealistic fears and phobias; psychoeducation in effective psychosocial coping techniques; and social therapy for them and their families aimed at improving their social supports. The hypothesis was that these additional services would result in experimental groups' functioning significantly better than comparison groups who did not receive the combination of skills training, social therapy, and psychotropic medications.

Treatment utilized behavioral techniques, including sessions for learning, review, rehearsal, and practice of the new coping skills patients were learning. Patients and their families in the experimental groups learned techniques for communicating better, asserting, enjoying leisure, reducing stress, conferring, planning, obtaining advice, solving personal problems, extinguishing phobias, controlling anxiety, depression, and impulsiveness, and enhancing social skills, as well as for building social supports with helpful friends and family.

Hypothesis for VA geographic unitization study with veteran psychiatric patients

Observed relation studies conducted with veteran psychiatric patients in the early 1970s assessed the special needs of these "orbiting" veteran patients. They were characterized as rootless, alienated from their families and home communities, and unable or unwilling to maintain stable employment and remain in a community.

Based on the findings of the assessments, observed causal studies hypothesized that migratory veteran psychiatric patients (as well as some native ones) would improve functionally with a treatment program that included efforts at helping them settle down and plant roots in a community where they could develop social supports and obtain continuity of care (R. E. Gordon, Lyons et al., 1973; R. E. Gordon & Webb, 1975). The studies and recommendations influenced the psychiatric staff at the veterans' hospital to unitize the hospital's program geographically and to establish outlying psychiatric aftercare clinics in the communities served by the hospital.

In the unitization program, all patients from a given geographic area were treated by the same staff of professionals both as inpatients and outpatients. If a patient was discharged from inpatient care, professionals who knew him in the hospital managed his outpatient care. If he returned to the hospital, they continued to treat him as an inpatient. Thus the staff came to know their patients well and to provide continuity of care to them and their families. Patients also benefited from getting to know other patients from their home communities with whom they could socialize and provide mutual support. This study, therefore, followed up on the social support component of the combined treatment research.

Hypothesis for modular psychoeducational treatment study of chronically ill mental hospital patients

Most chronic psychiatric patients, unlike typical medical patients with uncomplicated pneumonia or surgical ones with acute appendicitis, do not return to a previously high level of social functioning when they recover from the acute phase of their mental illnesses. Many never attained high levels previously. Theirs is not just a biomedical problem of neurotransmitters suddenly gone savagely awry, but one of multiple chronic defects – in coping skills and environmental supports as well as in psychophysiological condition (R. E. Gordon & Gordon, 1985). Thus, most chronic mental patients require special training in building coping skills and obtaining social supports.

The innovative feature of this new program for chronic mental patients, which was conducted in the late 1970s and early 1980s, was its use of psychoeducational modules to help repair their coping-skill defects and thus to enhance traditional state hospital psychiatric care. The modules were similar to those used in formal educational settings, but focused on training the psychosocial coping skills shown in Table 6.1. This table presents the kinds of skills taught in classes to patients of different ages and their families (R. E. Gordon & Gordon, 1981).

At the time this study was conducted we exercised some control over the resources of a state psychiatric treatment facility that cared for groups of chronically ill mental patients in the age categories child, adolescent, young adult, and elderly. Thus we could design programs to meet each group's needs and study their effectiveness. However, both ethical and political pressures interfered with the conduct of fully controlled experimental research with all the age groups. Only some of the components of each experiment could be controlled. Specifically, the research tested the effectiveness of each module with small matched experimental and control groups of patients. But no control unit was available where a ran-

Table 6.1. *Coping skills taught with psychoeducational modules in classes to groups of chronic mental patients of different ages and their families*

Category of skills	Components	Elderly	Young adults	Chronic adults	Adolescents	Children	Families
Survival skills	Medication training	X	X	X			X
	Personal information	X				X	
	Compliant behavior	X	X	X	X	X	X
Daily living skills	Personal hygiene/ eating/toilet	X		X	X	X	X
	Home care	X	X	X	X	X	X
	Independent living	X	X	X	X		
Personal/social skills	Managing stress		X	X			
	Communicating	X	X	X	X	X	X
	Personal health	X	X	X	X		
	Problem solving	X	X	X	X		X
	Asserting	X	X	X	X		X
	Negotiating		X		X		X
	Relaxing	X	X				X
	Sex role		X		X		
	Peer support		X	X	X		X
	Leadership		X				
Academic/vocational skills		X	X	X	X	X	
Leisure skills		X	X	X	X	X	X
Self-integrative skills	Building self-esteem	X					
	Clarifying values		X		X		X
	Goal setting		X	X			
	Measuring personal achievement				X		
Cognitive skills	Managing anxiety and depression	X	X	X			X

domly selected group of patients would receive only traditional psychiatric care at the treatment facility; all patients admitted to the treatment facility received treatment with the modular approach (plus traditional psychiatric care).

The hypothesis was that psychoeducational modules administered by ward paraprofessional staff under professional supervision would significantly improve the psychosocial skills and the functional level of chronically ill psychiatric patients who received them. This research carried forward the coping-skill training component of the combined treatment research.

Selecting subjects and designing the research

After making a hypothesis in an observed causal research, you need to find a large enough group of patients on whom to conduct your research. You need to match your groups so as to eliminate as many extraneous variables as possible. To do so, obtain demographic, health, and other information about your treatment and comparison groups of patients in order to determine whether the groups are well matched and to identify who is responding to your research treatment. You also need to standardize your research procedures.

All three studies, the combined treatment, VA geographic unitization, and modular psychoeducational programs, included every patient treated in the specific program during the period of the research. In these observed causal studies the selection of patients could not be controlled by random assignment to a treatment or control group, since it was necessary to treat all comers. However, comparison groups were used in all three studies. The section that follows shows what groups were used for comparison and how well the research and comparison groups matched each other in demographic, health, and other important characteristics.

The *combined treatment studies* retrospectively reviewed the office records of 810 private adult psychiatric outpatients treated in the 1950s. During this period major psychotropic medications and behavior management therapies were being introduced. Table 6.2 shows how the patients fell into four approximately equal-sized groups related to the kinds of treatment they received:

1. The first comparison group of patients were treated before major psychotropic medications and techniques from social learning theory and behavior therapy were available; they received only dynamic psychotherapy, minor tranquilizers, and referral for more heroic inpatient and shock treatments.

2. The first research group received major tranquilizers if they needed them, plus the dynamic therapy and minor tranquilizers that the first group obtained.

3. The second research group received behavior management and the combination of social-skills training and social therapy, in addition to the treatments the first two groups were getting.

4. The last research group received all of the therapies above plus antidepressants if they were depressed.

Demographic studies indicated that the four groups were well matched in terms of percentages of male and female, younger and older, married and unmarried, and richer and poorer patients. Table 6.2 also shows that all groups in the combined treatment study were similar in severity of illness in that each contained 15–16% of seriously emotionally ill patients who previously had required inpatient hospital care for their psychiatric illnesses. All four groups also included approximately 70% of patients who required only the psychosocial therapies – dynamic, behavioral, and social-support building – along with minor tranquilizers. In each group approximately 30% of patients required primarily medical

Table 6.2. Findings from observed causal research on combined psychiatric treatment, comparing the effectiveness of dynamic psychotherapy alone and in combination with psychotropic medications, social therapy, and behavior management techniques, in reducing private psychiatric outpatients' need for hospitalization and electroconvulsive therapy

| | | | Type of care required | | | | |
| | | | More intrusive or restrictive care | | Outpatient care | | |
Treatment introduced	No. of patients	Percentage of patients hospitalized previously	Inpatient hospitalization N (%)	Electroconvulsive therapy N (%)	Psychological treatment plus major psychotropics N (%)	Psychological treatment plus minor tranquilizers N (%)	Total (%)
(1) Dynamic psychotherapy alone	115	15	25 (22)	9 (8)	0 (0)	81 (70)	100
(1) Dynamic psychotherapy (2) Major tranquilizers	246	16	42 (17)	5 (2)	34 (14)	165 (67)	100
(1) Dynamic psychotherapy (2) Major tranquilizers (3) Skills and support training	217	16	20 (9)	2 (1)	43 (20)	152 (70)	100
(1) Dynamic psychotherapy (2) Major tranquilizers (3) Skills and support training (4) Antidepressants	232	16	16 (7)	0 (0)	53 (23)	163 (70)	100
Total (mean %)	810	16	249 (30)			561 (70)	100

Note: Comparing numbers of patients who required four levels of care – inpatient care, electroconvulsive therapy, major psychotropic medications, or psychotherapy and minor psychotropics – who were treated with each of the four different therapeutic approaches, chi-square = 61.3; 6 df; $p < .001$ (see Appendix Table A.1).

treatments – inpatient psychiatric hospitalization, electroconvulsive therapy (ECT), and/or major psychotropic medications.

In the *geographic unitization study,* every one of the 2,893 VA patients treated in the period 1969 to 1972 (before geographic unitization) and in 1974 (after unitization) was included. The preunitization patients served as a comparison group for the post unitization patients.

Follow-up interviews were conducted in the homes of 124 patients, 61 from the preunitization era and 63 from the postunitization period. There were no significant differences between the two cohorts of interviewed patients in age, sex, race, years of schooling, and highest educational degree attained. However, the preunitization group were more likely to be married, and the postunitization group to be black, single or divorced, and Vietnam veterans.

The *modular psychoeducational treatment study* compared elderly patients who entered the new program with those who turned down the opportunity. From among those hospitalized at a state hospital for an average of two years, 129 elderly patients were selected because they had no incapacitating physical illnesses. Seventy volunteered to be transferred to the research program. Fifty-nine, who remained in the traditional psychiatric program, became a comparison group. The groups were well matched on demographic and diagnostic data.

Deciding on measures and indicants of therapeutic outcome

Before you can evaluate the effectiveness of a program, you must find objective, valid, and reliable measures or indicants of outcome. Use different kinds of measures: physical, physiological, and biochemical when possible (with psychosomatic diseases like ulcer or hypertension, for instance), and standardized psychosocial measures, indicators of life adjustment in jobs, marriage, and the like, and attitude scales both with patients and significant others who know them well. The three studies provide you with examples of some of the measures and indicants that can be used for evaluating the effectiveness of a new program.

The *combined treatment study* used data-collection forms that were developed and routinely administered to all our private-practice patients in the 1950s and early 1960s, when these studies were conducted. These instruments were similar to the maternity questionnaire; they were based on findings from needs assessment research and provided information on patients' demographic and life-stress characteristics that appeared to be related to their psychiatric distress and their response to treatment. The posttreatment data forms included a number of objective measures of patients' functional level. The measures asked: Did the patient (1) require hospitalization or rehospitalization in a psychiatric facility? (2) continue or terminate marriage? (3) return to high school or college or remain a dropout? (4) receive or not receive new arrests and convictions for unlawful behavior? (5) obtain a better or worse job, keep the same one, lose it, or remain unemployed? (6) require shorter- or longer-term treatment? (7) need electroconvulsive therapy?

The VA *geographic unitization study* used other objective measures of the effectiveness and efficiency of treatment: (1) numbers of veteran patients receiving treatment; (2) average length of hospitalization; (3) percentage of recidivism; (4) percentage of referrals for aftercare; (5) level at which patient was functioning in the community and in the home; (6) level at which patient was functioning at work; (7) number of patients arrested; (8) efficiency of staff utilization; (9) treatment costs per patient.

These measures provide objective criteria by which to measure the outcome of geographic unitization that are important to the VA and the veteran patient population. A behavioral rating scale, the Katz Adjustment Scale (Katz & Lyerly, 1963), which had become available in the 1960s, was used to assess the postdischarge behavior and functioning of the VA patients.

The *modular psychoeducational-treatment program* employed a number of other behavioral rating scales. Some of these had become available during the 1960s to measure the effectiveness of drug studies. The measures included the following: (1) Nurses' Observational Scale for Inpatient Evaluation (NOSIE-30) (Honigfeld, Gillis & Klett, 1966); (2) Community Adjustment Potential (CAP) scale of the Discharge Readiness Inventory (Hogarty & Ulrich, 1972); (3) Social Adjustment Behavior Rating Scale (SABRS) (Aumack, 1962); (4) STAI (Spielberger, 1968); and others, including specific scales developed to assess progress in learning to perform the behaviors taught in each module (Patterson, 1982; Price & Moos, 1975).

The program also used other objective measures posttreatment appropriate to this population of elderly chronically ill patients in state mental hospitals: (1) length of hospital stay; (2) percentage discharged from hospital care to a community residence; (3) recidivism rate; (4) questionnaire responses regarding satisfaction with treatment and with new life situation.

Likert scales measured patients' and their friends' and families' responses. Likert scales are very commonly used to measure opinions and attitudes. They are made up of items with gradations of response along a single dimension – for example, the subject indicates strong agreement, agreement, indecision, disagreement, or strong disagreement with a given statement.

Determining what other resources are needed

The more complicated your study and the more outside people you need to employ, the more likelihood that it will be costly. As mentioned before, you can conduct the least expensive research with your own office patients.

The combined treatment study did just that; it involved only your own office and patients, cost nothing, and required no extra resources besides our family's efforts.

The VA geographic unitization study needed interviewers to visit discharged VA patients in their homes, some of which were over 60 miles from the hospital. Therefore, it required the hiring of interviewers, a part-time secretary, a part-time supervisor, and travel and computer time. The total cost was $10,000 spent over a period of one year. It was covered by a grant from the Veterans Administration.

The modular psychoeducational treatment program was conducted with the staff at a state mental institution. The overall cost per patient was approximately the same as that for patients who received routine care in the state institutions at the time – about $35 per day. The staff developed the modules, kept the research records, analyzed the data, and wrote a book about their findings (Patterson, 1982).

Collecting and analyzing data

You must plan in advance to collect and analyze data. Again, the least expensive method is to do it yourself with your own patients, utilizing the help of your office staff. With standardized intake forms, treatment planning instruments, and outcome measures, you routinely gather information from your patients in the process of assessing and treating them. Then you can analyze the data in a few hours a week and report the findings. This was how the data of the combined treatment studies were collected and analyzed.

The four groups of patients in the combined treatment research differed strikingly in their response to therapy. Some of the findings are shown in Table 6.2.

Note that there was a perfect relationship between the number of new therapies and the overall response of the patients. (1) Adding major tranquilizers decreased the percentage of patients who needed hospitalization or electroconvulsive therapy (ECT) from 30% to 19%. (2) Including skills and supports training further reduced the need for heroic therapies to 10% of patients. (3) Introducing antidepressants ended patients' need for ECT and diminished still further the percentage requiring hospital psychiatric care.

These studies were among the first to show the benefits of eclectic psychiatric treatment combining psychodynamic, behavioral, psychopharmacological, and psychoeducational methods as compared with the use of these therapeutic methods independently. Furthermore, patients who continued to receive individual office treatment every six months after they had recovered from the acute phase of their psychiatric disorders functioned at a significantly higher level than did those who discontinued treatment after recovery. The former were significantly more likely to avoid psychiatric hospitalization and criminal recidivism; they also significantly improved their education and job situations (R. E. Gordon, 1966).

Data were collected in the geographic unitization study from files in VA medical record rooms and by summer students paid on a VA grant to visit patients in their homes. Members of our family conducted the data analysis.

Comparisons between postunitization and preunitization data showed that geographic unitization of the hospital was significantly associated with many desired outcomes. In each comparison that follows, the post unitization finding is reported first. (1) Numbers of patients receiving treatment: Numbers of admissions nearly quadrupled to 819 from 208. (2) Average length of hospitalization: Decreased to 33 days from 57 days. (3) Readmissions: Despite the decreased length of hospital stay, percentage of readmissions remained fairly constant. (4) Referral for aftercare: 55% of discharged patients were referred as compared to 36% ($p < .001$). (5) Getting along with family: 80% of the patients reported that

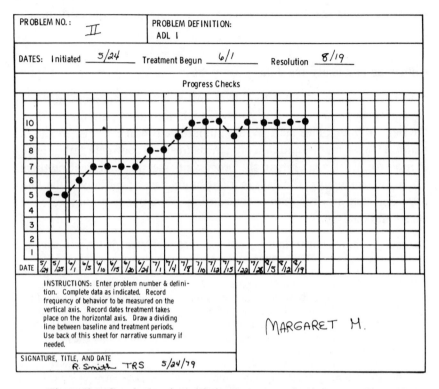

Figure 6.1. Graph showing a patient's progress in treatment. The patient's baseline level in performing basic living activities appears on the left side of the curve. The graph shows how her treatment continued until her performance stabilized.

they were getting along better, as compared to 42% (χ^2 = 4.1; $p < .05$). (6) Relationships with fellow workers and supervisors: Among patients who held jobs, 55% stated that they enjoyed favorable relationships, as compared to 17% (χ^2 = 5.4; $p < .02$). (7) Arrests: 22% of patients were arrested in comparison with 57% previously (χ^2 = 6.4; $p < .02$). (8) Utilization and cost of treatment staff: The treatment program utilized staff more efficiently after unitization, since the same staff were treating nearly four times as many patients; thus costs per patient decreased.

This research was one of the early studies that showed that the functioning of patients in a geographic unitization group was significantly improved over that of a preunitization group. Furthermore, it was cost-efficient.

Patient progress in the modular psychoeducational research program was measured both for each module and also on the standardized global rating scales mentioned previously in this chapter – the NOSIE-30, SABRS, and CAP scales. Paraprofessional day treatment staff, in addition to their regular psychiatric duties, learned the content and taught the modules under professional supervision

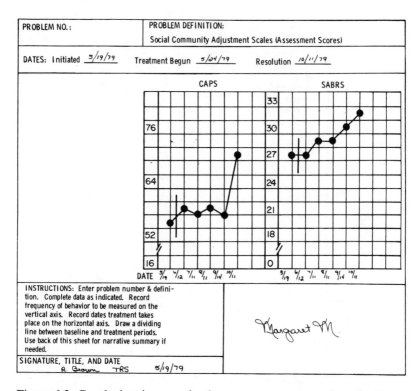

PROBLEM NO.:	PROBLEM DEFINITION:
	Social Community Adjustment Scales (Assessment Scores)

DATES: Initiated _3/19/79_   Treatment Begun _5/24/79_   Resolution _10/11/79_

INSTRUCTIONS: Enter problem number & definition. Complete data as indicated. Record frequency of behavior to be measured on the vertical axis. Record dates treatment takes place on the horizontal axis. Draw a dividing line between baseline and treatment periods. Use back of this sheet for narrative summary if needed.

SIGNATURE, TITLE, AND DATE
R. Brown   TRS   8/19/79

Figure 6.2. Graph showing a patient's progress as measured on the Community Adjustment Potential (CAP) scale and the Social Adjustment Behavioral Rating Scale (SABRS).

and scored the standardized rating scales. Night staff, in addition to their other duties, scored the day staff's ratings and helped keep the research records.

Figure 6.1 presents a graph of a patient's progress in modular basic living skills training, and Figure 6.2 her assessments on two global scales, the CAP and the SABRS (R. E. Gordon & Gordon, 1981). Each module was also individually evaluated in a causal relation experimental research, and was shown to be effective in achieving its goals. Figure 6.3 contains pooled data on 133 patients' improvement in coping as measured by the CAP and SABRS scales.

Plotting rating scale scores versus writing lengthy progress notes

Observe in Figures 6.1 and 6.2 how the graphic picture of rating scale scores shows at a glance whether a patient is making progress in psychiatric treatment. Compare these figures with temperature and blood pressure charts, where the same statement is true for patients receiving medical treatment for a fever or hypertension. Think about the hours you

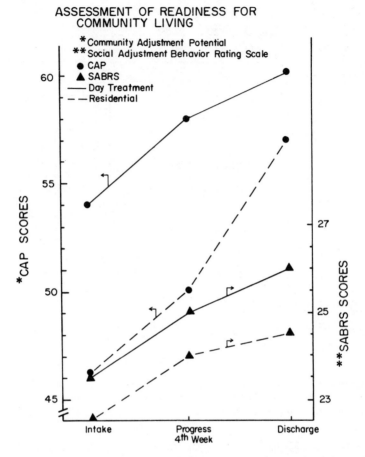

Figure 6.3. Graph presenting findings from an evaluation of a component of a psychoeducational treatment program. The table provides pooled data on 133 patients' progress. The patients' preparation for living in the community was assessed with the Social Adjustment Behavioral Rating Scale (SABRS) and the Community Adjustment Potential (CAP) scale.

have spent reading through voluminous pages of progress notes, and the time that you would have saved if the staff in the hospitals and clinics where your patients are being treated had put some of their time and energies into rating the patients and plotting their scores rather than just into recording the same thing verbally. Excellent software programs for the microcomputer exist for plotting graphs with data. The printed figures are suitable for publication.

Table 6.3. *Results of quasi-experimental observed causal study of the comparative effects of modular psychoeducational treatment upon the length of treatment, discharge rate, and rehospitalization rate of state mental hospital patients*

	Modular treatment	Traditional treatment
Number of patients	70	59
Effectiveness		
Mean length of stay before discharge (weeks)	17.2	21.7
Discharged from hospital (percentage)	74	53
Rehospitalization rates (percentage)	4	29

Note: As compared with patients who received only traditional psychiatric treatment, a significantly larger percentage of patients who received psychosocial skills training in modular classroom settings plus traditional psychiatric care were discharged ($x^2 = 13.5$; 1 df; $p < .001$). The latter patients required shorter stays in the hospital. Their rehospitalization rates were less than one-seventh of those of the comparison group ($x^2 = 10.1$; 1 df; $p < .01$).

Tables 6.3 and 6.4 compare outcome data of the modular psychoeducational and traditional psychiatric programs. Clearly, those receiving additional modular treatment were responding better to treatment than were those obtaining only traditional care. A year after discharge from the hospital, 77.4% of the elderly chronically ill mental patients who received modular psychoeducational treatment were still functioning at a higher level than were patients in the comparison group. They were living in homes throughout the community and were not clustered in slum neighborhoods. They were participating actively in social activities and leading lives of good quality. In contrast, only 23.9% of those treated by traditional methods were able to remain outside an institution.

Individual follow-up assessments after discharge of patients treated with the modular training approach showed that the patients had achieved their posthospitalization therapeutic goals. Table 6.4 contains some of the data.

Patients responded on a five-point Likert scale to the statement "My training prepared me to move into the community" with a range of responses from *strongly agree* = 1 to *strongly disagree* = 5. Their median response of 2.00 indicates substantial agreement. Relatives and friends rated the patients on their level of adjustment after completing the program. The five alternative responses ranged from *Worse now than she/he was before treatment* = 1, through *Somewhat better now than she/he was before treatment* = 3, to *Very much better now than she/he was before treatment* = 5. The median response was 4.0, which agreed with the alternative response *Much better now than she/he was before treatment* (Patterson, 1982).

Table 6.4. *Results of quasi-experimental observed causal study of the comparative effects of modular psychoeducational treatment upon the community placement of discharged patients*

Destination	Modular treatment (percentage)	Traditional treatment (percentage)
Independent living	23	7
Boarding or foster homes	30	5
Not discharged from hospital	26	47
Living with family	17	34
Other	4	7
Total	100	100

Note: Fewer patients who volunteered for modular treatment had families.

Seventy percent of the former state hospital patients who received modular psychoeducational coping-skills training were living in noninstitutional settings in the community after discharge, as compared with 46% of the comparison group ($x^2 = 7.76$; 1 *df*; $p < .01$).

Statistical analysis

You do not need complicated multivariate statistics to conduct research like these examples with your patients. All these studies used chi-square to analyze the significance of differences between research and comparison groups.

Writing up results

Problems with observed causal research

Reports of results of observed causal research must emphasize the problems in drawing more than observed relation conclusions from the findings. Many extrinsic factors besides treatment variables can bring about changes in patients' responses unless the researcher carefully prevents or controls them in designing the study.

The combined treatment studies leave a number of questions unanswered. Can you think of some of them? For example, could the results be related to our growing therapeutic experience over the period of eight years of the study and not specifically to the new behavioral, social support, and psychopharmacological therapies? Was the patient population changing as different types of patients began to seek help? Was there a changed community attitude, such as less stigma toward mental patients, that might have enabled patients in the later years to respond better to treatment than those who were treated earlier? Were the patient groups drawn from the same population in the three investigations? (They were not randomly assigned in advance to their respective experimental and comparison groups.) You must discuss these kinds of issues when reporting on the findings of your observed causal studies.

In the geographic unitization research, the hospital director might have decided to unitize the wards one by one, sending patients randomly first to the new unitized programs and then to the old-style units for treatment. If you ever have any administrative voice in a decision of this sort, use it. Only then can you properly infer causality from the new treatment's findings. However, since this was not done, we can state only that the new treatment was related to the improved outcomes. During the 1969 to 1974 period when unitization took place, other events were also occurring in the psychiatric community at large that may have affected psychiatric patients in veterans' hospitals and may have accounted for many of the results: (1) Many psychiatric hospitals throughout the country were treating a larger number of patients than they previously had been doing, but keeping them for shorter hospitalizations, a movement that may have influenced the first two results above, and (2) other new treatments – such as the psychopharmacological, behavior management, and psychoeducational therapies described in the other two researches – were being introduced, a fact that may have resulted in postunitization patients getting better therapy.

The modular psychoeducational research program contained a very important causal relation feature: It assessed the effectiveness of each individual psychoeducational module in controlled studies. Nevertheless, it left open the question whether the patients who did not volunteer for the new treatment, but chose to remain in the state hospital, would have responded as well to the psychoeducational approach. Were the volunteers the patients with a better prognosis initially? Or was the new research-unit setting truly responsible for the benefits observed?

To answer some of these questions, modular psychoeducational treatment was implemented with geriatric patients in another state institution. It produced similar improvements with the new patients, but there still were no matched controls. If you are ever in a position to evaluate the effectiveness of a new program, assign patients randomly to both the new program and to a traditional unit, and collect the same objective research data from both to compare the outcomes of the new and old treatment approaches. Then you can state with confidence whether the new treatment is more effective or not.

Publishing

The quasi-experimental program evaluations described here received greater credence because they were being preceded and followed up by related research, some of which was well controlled. They were accepted by publications because they were part of continuing studies. Related reports on patients' needs assessments and on controlled experimental studies were also appearing in the literature.

Summary

This chapter has described observed causal research. Three clinical program evaluations served to illustrate the conduct of this kind of study and some of the benefits and problems. The hypotheses for the research interventions grew out of earlier observed relation research findings of patients' characteristics and needs. Each of the three treatment programs was designed to improve patients' functioning. Since the Axis V scale was not yet available, other objective measures of patients' functioning were used to measure the dependent variable.

When you perform an observed causal relation research, give proper recognition to the limitations of your study in both the methods and discussion sections of your reports. Do your best to keep constant as many extraneous variables as possible. You may eventually get an opportunity to evaluate more fully the effectiveness of your new therapies in a better controlled experiment.

7. Causal relation research

As a researcher you have an obligation to conduct as rigorous a study as possible. This chapter shows how to select qualified subjects, carefully define your variables, and analyze your results. If you ever find yourself in a senior administrative position in a treatment facility, have the power to assign patients to the various treatment units, and are called upon to evaluate the effectiveness of a new treatment program, conduct a causal relations experiment. This chapter uses two causal relation studies to provide examples of the points made: (1) *preventing postpartum emotional distress* and (2) *reducing rehospitalization of state hospital patients by peer management and support.* Needs assessments of patients preceded both of these causal relation investigations.

Definition

A research has reached the causal relation stage if it fulfills the following criteria:

1. There are (at least) two measured variables.
2. The treatment (in the broad sense of the word) is applied to an experimental group of patients/subjects and withheld from a control group. Note that there may be two or more values of the treatment, as, for example, different dosages of the same drug. In this case, the treatment is called the *treatment variable.*
3. All possible relevant conditions other than the treatment are held constant so that the control group will be as much like the experimental group as possible, except for the treatment applied by the researcher. If this is done, then there is a high probability that any changes in the dependent variable for the experimental group can be attributed to the treatment.

4. There must be one or more dependent variables. The dependent variables are those that are observed by the researcher after the treatment is applied. They are measured in both the experimental and control groups to see if the experimental group showed a greater change than the controls.

Most causal relation research with psychiatric patients and other human subjects nowadays focuses only on therapy – on medicating or on preventing or reducing stress and other disease-causing conditions. It seeks to avoid causing or increasing pathogenic processes. Take, for instance the rape and rape-resister studies mentioned previously. How would you test the relative merits of resisting an attack when the rapist is armed with a gun, knife, or other weapon? Would you ask women of different ages and races to volunteer to expose themselves to dangerous situations where they might get raped and randomly select groups who would be instructed to resist and others not to resist? Such a study would be difficult to launch, to say the least.

Researchers do use animals to conduct causal relation experiments to test hypotheses about pathogenesis. You can create experimental neurosis-like or psychosis-like conditions in animals and try out the effects of various treatments upon them. This procedure is used regularly in the early stages of psychotropic and other drug research.

Making a hypothesis

As before, your first task in launching a causal relation research is to make a hypothesis. The two examples described in this chapter – preventing postpartum emotional distress and reducing rehospitalization of state hospital patients by peer management and support – built upon information obtained in studies that were mentioned in earlier chapters. These included the combined treatment, modular psychoeducational, and psychiatric maternity research, in particular. Data from needs assessments of the last group of studies, conducted with the maternity questionnaire, and from experience in treating them with the combined treatment approach provided ideas for the hypothesis of the research into preventing postpartum emotional distress. Further, knowledge gained from the findings of this preventive causal relation study, which was conducted in the late 1950s and early 1960s, was subsequently fed back into the clinical treatment program for perinatal women who sought psychiatric care. It also helped pave the way for the study into reducing rehospitalization.

Hypothesis for the study on preventing postpartum emotional distress

Studies of psychiatric maternity patients identified a number of life stresses that were highly correlated with women's emotional reactions during and after pregnancy. At the time of the studies in the 1950s, many young married couples had left their childhood homes, families, and friends and flocked to the nation's suburbs to raise their children. They did not realize that the women might be overstressing themselves with their new responsibilities, and might find themselves without social supports in a time of need, such as during the perinatal period (R. E. Gordon, Gordon & Gunther, 1961).

Until that period of the 1950s, psychiatrists and social scientists knew little about the importance to mental health of peer-group and other social supports. However, experience with the combined treatment approach, which included efforts at helping patients improve their social environmental supports and their coping skills, had been especially effective in helping perinatal women recover from their emotional illnesses. A factor-analytic observed relation study (see chapter 5) indicated that maternal stresses could be divided into two main factors, one related to personal insecurity arising out of traumata in the mother's personal background, and the other associated with conflict in her new maternal role related in part to her lack of adequate social support (R. E. Gordon, Kapostins & Gordon, 1965). The causal relation research was conducted to determine whether reducing stress and improving supports would reduce maternity patients' postpartum distress.

Women who were attending antenatal classes at the local community hospital participated in the study. It hypothesized that antenatal women who responded to instruction by making recommended changes to reduce stress in their lives, improve their coping skills, and increase their social supports would react significantly better emotionally in the postpartum period than would uninstructed controls (R. E. Gordon, 1961).

Hypothesis for research on reducing rehospitalization of state hospital patients by peer management and support

This research was performed in the late 1970s when we had some direction and control over a state mental hospital's treatment program. Information from the preventive work above as well as from the quasi-experimental combined treatment studies was used in a controlled therapeutic setting. Although random selection of inpatients to experimental and control groups in the treatment facility was not possible, this was not true with assignment for aftercare.

The reducing rehospitalization program was designed to augment the modular psychoeducational project described in the last chapter in a controlled causal relation research. Its research hypothesis was that patients who received the special psychoeducational coping-skill training plus social-support training and then joined a Community Network Development (CND) for discharged patients would function better in the community and require less rehospitalization than would a control group who received only skill training but were referred for standard psychiatric aftercare in the community.

144   Chapter 7

The Axis V scale was not yet available to measure patients' functional levels. Therefore other objective measures were used to assess the dependent variable. The modular psychoeducational project for chronically ill mental patients focused primarily on measuring the benefits of psychoeducational coping-skill training for chronic mental inpatients while they were residing in the hospital. The reducing rehospitalization project also provided coping-skill training and psychotropic medications to chronic mental patients, but it held these therapies constant. It investigated the effectiveness of teaching patients to make friends and build support groups with peers after they left the institution. It also developed a mutual support group for patients – the Community Network Development (CND) – which patients joined upon leaving the hospital (Edmunson, Bedell, Archer & Gordon, 1982; Edmunson, Bedell & Gordon, 1984; R. E. Gordon & Gordon, 1981).

The reducing rehospitalization program thus supplemented the modular psychoeducational one, focusing primarily on the issue of peer support. The combined treatment studies discussed in chapter 6 had pointed to possible benefits of mutual support to patients. The projects for reducing rehospitalization and preventing postpartum distress followed up by testing these benefits in causal relation research. The reducing rehospitalization study also served to evaluate the benefits of continuity of care provided by patients themselves and their peers.

Needs assessments conducted by Edmunson and others (R. E. Gordon, Edmunson, Archer & Weinberg, 1981), which compared psychiatric patients with better and worse social-supports networks, showed that (1) patients with poor social network supports and little reciprocity (mutual giving and receiving assistance between patients and their network members) were likely to require longer hospitalizations (r between strength of network and length of hospitalization = $-.33$; $p < .05$); (2) those with destructive networks (containing irritating persons who made patients feel worse or frustrated them) had greater numbers of arrests for criminal behavior ($r = .45$; $p < .0001$); (3) those with positive and warm feelings toward network members had fewer arrests ($r = -.26$; $p < .04$) and were less likely to attempt suicide ($r = .36$; $p < .004$); while (4) those with irritating persons in their networks were more likely to make suicide attempts ($r = .40$; $p < .001$). These findings provided some information on what the patients' special training sessions should cover – special preparation for making friends, providing reciprocal support, and community living as members of a patient support group.

Deciding on subjects/patients

Random selection

To run a clinical causal relation experiment, you randomly select patients/subjects with a known quality (such as a disease condition), treat these subjects in some manner you think will affect that quality, and then test to see if you made a change in it (cured the disease). But how can you be sure that the change you find was due to the treatment you administered? You can never be absolutely certain. But you can state with a high probability that this was the case if you control other variables – such as psychiatric diagnosis (*DSM-III* Axes I and II), other medical diagnoses (Axis III), aggravating stresses (Axis IV scores), premorbid functional level (Axis V score), sex, age, socioeconomic position, race, religion, education, and marital status – that might affect the outcome of your research.

You do this by randomly selecting another sample of subjects from the same population with that same known quality, letting the same period of time elapse, and then testing them to see if the quality changed when no experimental treatment was administered.

If your second group was not much like the first, then you still cannot say much about what caused the results. For this reason, your second group should be as much like the first as possible; this is why we specified in the preceding paragraph that they should be taken "from the same population." Recall the discussion about samples and populations (see chapter 3): If your experimental group consists of 10 primiparas between the ages of 21 and 30, living within a certain catchment area, and of mixed ethnic group, then your control group should have those same qualities. To control in an experiment means "to hold constant." Thus you are controlling for the variables of age, sex, number of pregnancies, geographic area, ethnicity, and so on, because these variables are approximately the same (i.e., approximately "constant") in both groups. In other words, you must try to control those that you do not wish to vary and study. How you go about doing this is explained in the sections that follow.

The reason for paying attention to random selection of your subjects is that all the statistics you will use are based upon the assumption of randomly selected cases. To the extent that you violate this assumption, you are threatening the validity of your results. Obviously, if your selection of subjects is heavily biased in any direction, your results will have little or no validity.

Random assignment

This was the approach used in both the studies described below. You select a pool of similar subjects twice as large as you intend your experimental group to be. You then randomly assign each subject to either the experimental or the control group. Often you can make a random assignment by providing your treatment and control procedures with numbers from 0 to 9. For example, if you had two treatment groups and a control,

Treatment A could get numbers 1–3, B could get 4–6, and the controls could get 7–9. Then, using a table of random numbers, you assign each patient/subject from the population to the appropriate treatment group. In this way, you insure that both groups came from the same population. Then you administer your treatment to the experimental group, while exposing the control group to all the same conditions (including elapsed time, attention) except the treatment. Later you test both groups to determine if any changes in the known quality they all started with were significantly larger in the experimental group (who received the treatment) than in the control group (who did not receive the treatment).

Matching

You may exercise even greater control over these variables by matching each subject in your experimental group with one in the control group. Randomly select subjects for your experimental group; then selectively match a group of control subjects to them. This requires that you decide ahead of time what the important variables are: for example, age, sex, socioeconomic status. For each experimental subject, find a control subject who matches on these variables. Thus, if you have a 37-year-old woman of Irish extraction in the experimental group, you will need a 37-year-old woman of Irish extraction in the control group, and so on for each patient. This is a *matched control* group.

When you start your experiment, your 20 subjects are all from the same population – the population you define when you describe their characteristics. You administer your treatment to the experimental group, and retest both experimental and control groups. In all other respects, the two groups are the same, the only difference being that the experimentals received the treatment and the controls did not. If you find a statistical difference between the groups in the magnitude of the original known quality (anxiety, for example), you can conclude that there is a high probability that it was your treatment that made the difference.

All controls are instituted for this purpose – to allow you to make convincing statements about the results you observe. To be convincing to the scientific community, these statements must be based upon recognized procedures for controlling the effects of variables.

In the study on preventing postpartum emotional distress, women attending antenatal classes were randomly assigned to be controls or experimentals. Altogether there were 85 experimentals and 76 controls. The groups were subdivided into control and experimental classes for couples, where both members of a couple attended, and control and experimental classes for wives, where only the wife attended.

Controlling for passage of time in research

With the passage of time, many factors outside the treatment situation may intervene to affect patients' behavior and interfere with a research. You control this problem by conducting your experiment with both controls and experimentals at the same time. However, in clinical settings it often takes time to collect an adequate sample of patients for your experimental and control groups. In the study on preventing postpartum distress, it took a year to obtain enough women in antenatal classes to provide experimental and control groups. This meant that participants in the second half of the year might pick up information by word of mouth about the content of the instructions from participants in the first half, since it was impossible to prevent their meeting and talking with each other. The experiment was therefore designed in advance to make use of this important variable. Both experimental and control patients were subdivided into those who participated in the first half of the year and those who attended classes in the second half of the year.

Altogether, this gave eight research subgroups for the study on preventing postpartum emotional distress, as shown in Table 7.1. There were four groups each of experimentals who attended special classes and controls who received only traditional antenatal training. Among these, approximately half of the subjects participated in the first half of the experiment. And in approximately half of the groups, the wives attended classes alone, while half came with their husbands. The table shows how the independent variable was ranked by the amount of exposure to the special instructions that each group of women received. This was an advantage to the research, since it provided a method of grading the amount of exposure to instructions that each group received and thus of putting the independent variable on an ordinal scale.

In the research on reducing rehospitalization of state hospital patients, a group of 80 patients were randomly divided into two groups of 40 patients each. For the last three weeks of the nine-week period of modular psychoeducational treatment in the hospital, both continued to receive the skill-building treatment. The experimentals additionally joined a network of discharged psychiatric outpatients who now lived in the community – the Community Network Development (CND) – where they learned peer support, counseling, and group-leadership skills. The controls continued to attend only regular psychoeducational classes during the three-week period.

At the end of a total of nine weeks of treatment, both the experimental peer-support group and the control group were discharged from the hospital. Appointments for aftercare were made for the controls at the community mental health clinics near their homes. The experimentals continued to participate in the CND, led by four patients who served as peer leaders.

Table 7.1. *Outline of causal relation procedure used in the research on preventing postpartum distress*

Subjects[a]	Period in study	Filled in Q_1	Rank of independent variable	Mediating variable (filled in Q_2)	Dependent variable (judged emotional reaction)	
					6 wk.	6 mo.
Experimental wives' classes	1st half	Yes	4	Yes	Yes	Yes
	2nd half	Yes	3	Yes	Yes	No
Experimental couples' classes	1st half	Yes	1	Yes	Yes	Yes
	2nd half	Yes	1	Yes	Yes	No
Control wives' classes	1st half	Yes	7	Yes	Yes	Yes
	2nd half	Yes	5	Yes	Yes	No
Control couples' classes	1st half	Yes	7	Yes	Yes	Yes
	2nd half	Yes	5	Yes	Yes	No

Subjects: Groups of randomly selected expectant wives attending antenatal classes alone (wives' classes) or with their husbands (couples' classes), matched by background questionnaire data (Q_1).
Independent variable: Exposure to experimental class instructions. Measured by ranked amount of exposure to the instructional information.
Mediating variable: Subjects' behavioral response. Measured by verbal responses of subjects on the follow-up questionnaire (Q_2).
Dependent variable: Subjects' postnatal emotional reaction. Measured by physicians' and nurses' judgments.
[a]Subjects who delivered in the first six months of the experiment were included in the first-half groups; the remainder were placed in the second-half groups.

Deciding what test instruments are needed

You need to select instruments for assessing your independent variable (the existing known condition to which you intend to apply a treatment) and your dependent variable(s) (the quality(ies) that you expect to be affected by the treatment you impose). You must have a standard, or at least a uniform, test to show the results. This means, at the very least, that a set of scores is obtained from all subjects in the same way under the same conditions. Ideally, the test will be written so that other experimenters at any other locations could apply it to their groups of similar subjects by following the instructions that are supplied with it.

Here again, if a test that meets your needs has already been published, by all means use it, since you will then avoid the time and expense inherent in constructing a new instrument. Your test need not get into such problems at all if you intend to look at easily recognizable standards of performance such as "abstaining from alcohol for more than one year," "maintaining a perfect attendance record at school," or "eliminating enuresis." However, even using criteria like these, you need to make up data-collection forms for recording the results you expect after administering your treatment.

In some experiments there is more than one dependent variable. In other words, you may expect the treatment you apply to affect more than one quality in your subjects. (In many experiments there is also more than one independent variable.)

In the research on preventing postpartum emotional distress, all the patients, both experimentals and controls, filled in the maternity questionnaire (Q_1 in Table 7.1). Experimentals and controls were similar on all the variables that predict perinatal emotional distress, except that more controls had failed to complete their education.

After delivery, the women filled in the postnatal version of the maternity questionnaire while still in the maternity ward of the hospital. It provided information on the changes they had made in their lives since they filled in the first questionnaire; this was the *mediating variable* (Q_2 in Table 7.1).

After the maternity patients returned to their homes, their obstetricians and the hospital public health nurses rated their postnatal emotional distress on a five-point scale – the *dependent variable*. These ratings took place at the time of their routine follow-up examinations – six weeks and six months after delivery. Thus no special effort or cost was needed to obtain ratings of the patients' emotional condition.

The peer leaders in the investigation into reducing rehospitalization filled in *Likert scales,* which were used to determine the level of stress and/or reward they felt, the significance of their peer-management job in their lives, and their self-perception of their performance in the job (see chapter 6).

Designing the study

In some studies you must be concerned about the effects of the patients' earlier experience in the experiment. These arise in drug studies, where the effects of a drug can influence later performance.

Drug studies

In a trial of several different drugs with long-lasting effects, you cannot give more than one experimental drug or medicine to the same patients. You must follow the same kind of design as with the maternity patients in the study on preventing postpartum emotional distress and randomly assign different patients to experimental and control groups.

You can, however, use the same patients as their own controls with medicines whose effects wear off rapidly. You must be certain that the time between administering the first drug is sufficiently long for all of its effects to have disappeared before you administer the second drug. Otherwise, you will actually be measuring some residual effects of the first drug instead of the effects of the second drug alone. To be able to use patients as their own controls is a major advantage in research; you save both time and money, since you need to recruit and pay for only half as many patients for the study.

Remember to think about what extraneous factors can possibly contaminate your study, and either control for them or eliminate them by the way you design your research. Two kinds of designs allow you to assign each drug and level of dosage to every patient: the *randomized block* and the *Latin square*.

Randomized block design

In a randomized block design each subject is used as his or her own control for each experimental procedure, but the order of presentation of each procedure is randomized over subjects to avoid effects of using each treatment first, second, and so on. This *crossover* design has many advantages, chiefly that the effect of differences between patients is minimal. It also allows the use of fewer patients, because several measures are obtained on each one. However, there are a number of stipulations as to when and how the randomized block design should be used, and the interpretations of the experimental results must be subjected to an *analysis of variance*.

Latin square design

The Latin square design is similar to the randomized block design but makes it possible to extract even more information from the data you obtain from your research subjects. It is particularly useful where the research is costly in terms of time or money. Like use of the randomized block design, use of the Latin square design and the related *Greco-Latin Square* involves making several assumptions about the type of observations you collect. If these assumptions are not warranted, then the sophisticated design will only obscure the significance of your results rather than enhancing them. These data, too, must then be subjected to an analysis of variance for interpretation of the results. The services of a consultant should be retained to assist in these designs and analyses.

Analysis of variance (ANOVA) designs

Analysis of variance (often abbreviated as ANOVA) is a method for looking at experimental results from more than two groups at a time. It encompasses many different designs, some of them complex, for getting the maximum amount of information out of the smallest number of subjects. It also allows you to perform a series of treatments in the course of one experiment rather than making only one change in your independent variable to determine whether or not it results in a change in your dependent variable. The following will give a brief overview of the procedure and rationale for setting up a multivariate experiment and subjecting it to an analysis of variance.

When we apply a *t* test, the purpose is to compare one mean with another. Our research hypothesis is: Mean 1 is not the same as Mean 2; and our null hypothesis is: Mean 1 = Mean 2, or "There is no significant difference between Mean 1 and Mean 2."

However, we may wish to test more than one mean against another. Select a random sample of, say, 40 patients, measure them all on some variable, then divide them in half and subject 20 of them to Treatment X. This is your experimental group. The other 20 (who do not get the treatment) constitute your control group. You administer Treatment X because you believe that it will cause a change in another variable, *Y*. Then you measure *Y* in both your experimental group and your control group. If your *t* test shows that the mean *Y* in the experimental group is significantly different from that in the control group (and all other variables have been handled appropriately), you can conclude that your administration of Treatment X was responsible for this change in Y in the experimental group.

However, suppose that Treatment X is a drug for inducing sleep in insomniacs. You may know that the drug has a positive effect on sleep, and you may know the maximum amount to administer to avoid harmful effects. But you do not know the optimum amount simply to induce a restful night's sleep. It would be wasteful and costly in time, as well as other resources, to continually draw a sample of subjects, divide them in half, and compare them with each other. A more efficient method would be to draw a larger sample, divide them into several groups, and administer the drug to each group in a different strength. For example, Group 1 might receive 1 mg (call this Treatment X_1); the second group, 3 mg (call this Treatment X_2); the third group, 5 mg (call this Treatment X_3); and the fourth group, 10 mg (call this Treatment X_4).

The Y variable – the one you hope will be positively affected by your administration of the drug – will be "amount of deep sleep during a specified eight-hour period." (This assumes, of course, that you have operationally defined "deep sleep" as a specific configuration of EEG waves taken during the designated sleep period.)

Your research hypothesis may be that the mean Y for the group receiving Treatment X_1 will be less than the mean Y for the group receiving Treatment X_2, which will be less than the mean Y for the group receiving Treatment X_3, which will be less than the mean Y for the group receiving Treatment X_4.

Or, if you are not sure that you will always get positive results (that is, increased sleep) as you increase the dosage, your research hypothesis will be that each mean Y will be different from the other mean Y's. We can write this in symbols as:

$$MY_1 \neq MY_2 \neq MY_3 \neq MY_4$$

Your null hypothesis will be:

$$MY_1 = MY_2 = MY_3 = MY_4$$

where M refers to the mean of each experimental group.

The experiment above is a typical case where you would use ANOVA to compare the results of all these treatments at the same time. Your independent variables are the treatments, that is, the different dosages of the drug. The resulting measurements of Y (sleeping time for each group) are measures of the dependent variable. These are called *treatment effects*.

There will be some variability within each of the groups, and you hope that there will be some variability between groups. (If not, you will not know the optimum dosage to increase the amount of sleep of your insomniacs.) At the same time, if there is so much variability within each group that it is as large as the variability between the groups, you still will not know the optimum dosage.

Therefore, a measure is needed to show that the variability between groups is greater than the variability within groups. This measure is called the F test. It is the ratio of the mean sum of squares between groups to the mean sum of squares within groups. (It can be shown mathematically that each of these mean squares is a measure of variance.) As this ratio grows larger than 1, you will be able to say with a higher degree of confidence (ergo, a lower probability of chance results) that the group means are significantly different from each other. The results of your research would then be that there is a high probability that increasing the dosage causes an increase in the (defined) type of sleep. Within the structure of the ANOVA design, there are further tests that you can perform to show which dosage is causing the largest positive effect.

The F test is a parametric test for the analysis of variance. If your measures (either of the treatment or of its possible effects) do not meet the requirements for a parametric test, then you should use either the Friedman two-way analysis of variance, or the Kruskal–Wallis one-way analysis of variance.

Using a research or statistical consultant

When using complicated design and statistical analyses like the one above, you should consult a professional statistician or consultant in research design. Otherwise, you may use an inappropriate statistic with your data and thus may obtain meaningless results.

If you foresee a problem in the design of your study and choice of statistic, you should obtain a consultant early, as soon as you have outlined your hypothesis, subjects, and proposed procedure, and before you have begun to collect any data. A consultant will assist you in designing your study, determining the size of your sample, selecting your patients and controls, and choosing your statistic, as well as in other ways.

After your consultation you can proceed on your own in collecting the data, plugging them into your computer program, and analyzing them. If you do this yourself with your office staff, your family, and your microcomputer, your costs will only be for your and their time and a modest fee for the consultant. You can discuss your findings periodically with your consultant and obtain guidance with a problem.

On the other hand, you can ask your consultant to handle the management of the data and perform the statistical analysis for you. Then you will need to pay for the time required. Finally, the statistician or research design expert may become a full collaborator in your research, participating in developing hypotheses, reading the literature, writing reports, and all other phases of the work.

Psychosocial research

In experimental psychosocial research with psychiatric patients:

1. Assess the effects of the *independent variable* upon the *mediating variable,* if there is one, and those of the *mediating variable* upon the *dependent variable.* If you told us only that you can reach out with your hand and make water flow, we might think that you can work magic. However, if you stated that you reached out, took hold of a mediating device – a water faucet – and turned your wrist, we should understand better how you made the water flow. Further, it would be helpful if you showed that a 45-degree turn resulted in a slight flow, a 90-degree turn in a greater flow, and a 180-degree turn in a still greater rush of water. The situation is the same in psychiatry.

Showing only that psychotherapy helps patients without explaining specifically what you do, how the patients change their behavior as a result, and what happens to their emotional state is not very convincing to skeptics. They are more convinced when they know the details of your interventions and what your patients did because of them. In the modular psychoeducational treatment study, the modules used with the geriatric patients were clearly described and the method of their use explained. The research on preventing postpartum emotional distress described below provides explicit details as to the independent variable (the specific and detailed experimental instructions the patients heard), the mediating variable (the number and kinds of changes the patients made), and the dependent variable (a quantified measure of the subsequent emotional response of the patients).

2. Control for the *placebo effect.* Since patients will respond to attention alone, you must control for the fact that patients are included in a study even when they do not receive any active treatment. In both the research on preventing postpartum emotional distress and on reducing rehospi-

talization, the control groups spent exactly the same amount of time receiving instructions as did the experimentals. The women in antenatal classes in the former study attended extra sessions on routine infant care topics; in the latter research, the control group of 40 chronic mental patients received extra modular psychoeducational coping-skill classes during the last three weeks of their hospitalizations at the same time as the experimentals received training in peer management and support.

In drug studies, the placebo effect is controlled by giving patients a harmless, inactive substance that looks no different from the active medicines being tested. It is included in the experimental design in exactly the same manner as are the active experimental drugs.

3. When studying the effects of a new therapy, control for the possible effects of therapist personality, style, and other related extraneous variables by using a *crossover design,* as mentioned above in the paragraph on randomized block design. In this, therapists switch roles in the middle of the experiment; those who were treating experimentals now take over the controls; and those who were working with the controls switch to the experimentals. In the research on preventing postpartum emotional distress, the public health nurses who had taught the controls in the first period of the study subsequently took over the training of the experimentals.

4. Try whenever you can to *grade the amount of treatment* patients receive, and to measure the amount by which they respond or react to it. For example, rather than just giving a single dose of a drug or placebo, use a number of different dosages to determine which is the optimum.

In the combined treatment research described in chapter 6, patients received four different gradations of care, and a larger percentage reacted favorably as each new treatment step was added. Likewise, the research on preventing postpartum distress provided different levels of treatment to the eight groups. It measured both the groups' behavioral responses and their emotional reactions.

5. Keep the investigators, subjects, and evaluators *blind* as to whether subjects are experimentals or controls in order to avoid unconscious bias. In the maternity studies, neither the obstetrician judges nor the patients themselves were informed about the design of the experiments and which patients were experimentals or controls until the studies were completed. However, it is not possible to keep subjects and evaluators completely blind in this kind of psychosocial experiment, because in the group sessions the subjects can describe what went on. Anyone can then determine with a little probing who is an experimental or a control. This problem

need not arise in drug studies, where experimental and control drugs can be packaged to look exactly the same.

6. After the experimental procedure is completed, *compare the demographic and other important characteristics* of patients who benefit from treatment with those of patients who do not respond so well. This was done in the experiment on preventing postpartum emotional distress.

7. *Follow up* the study for five years, if possible. Longitudinal studies that show whether the effects of an experimental condition remain after a considerable period of time are more believable than cross-sectional ones that just look at patients at a single point in time or for a short period. The study on preventing postpartum emotional distress carried out a five-year follow up.

The experimentals in the study on preventing postpartum emotional distress received special instructions while the controls were attending extra sessions of standard prenatal class instruction. The information provided in the instructions was derived from prior observed relation and observed causal research with maternity and other psychiatric patients. The instructions were these: (1) Seek help and take advice while you're learning to be a mother. (2) Make friends with couples who are more experienced than you are with babies and little children. (3) Don't overload yourself with tasks that are less important than mothering. (4) Don't be too concerned with how your home looks. (5) Get plenty of rest and sleep. (6) Don't be a nurse to elderly relatives during this maternity period. (7) Talk over your worries with your doctor, husband, family, and friends. (8) Keep up your outside interests but cut down on your participation. (9) Arrange for baby-sitters in advance so you don't feel put out when you can't find one. (10) Learn to drive a car (if you don't know how already) so you and the baby won't be shut-ins. (11) If you've been thinking of moving into larger quarters, don't move now; wait until you've adjusted to being a mother.

As noted above, experimentals, controls, and their husbands who participated in the research in the first half of the year may have been exposed to more experimental information than women who participated in the second half of the year. Further, those who attended instruction sessions with their husbands were more likely to pick up points than those who attended alone. These considerations gave us a method of ranking the independent variable – the amount of exposure to instructions the women received in each of the eight groups of controls and experimentals – as shown in Table 7.1. We devised this method before the experiment began.

The new mothers' obstetricians and the public health nurses who visited them in their homes rated the women's postnatal emotional adjustment at six weeks and six months after delivery. This procedure provided the measure of the dependent variable. Each patient received two ratings. A correlation of .85 between the ratings showed a high degree of agreement between the raters on postnatal adjustment of the new wives. The entire research procedure is outlined in Table 7.1.

In the study on reducing rehospitalization, members of the Community Network Development (CND) met weekly for socializing as well as sessions of group problem solving. With the help of the patient group leaders they organized patient business, fund-raising, and leisure activities. They were encouraged to contact each other during the week for mutual support and assistance in managing problems.

Obtaining permission

The experimental and control patients in both studies needed to fill in informed-consent forms to participate in the experiment.

Determining what other resources are needed

In many clinical research situations, conducting causal relation research can be an expensive process. However, the costs of the study on preventing postpartum emotional distress were kept to a minimum because the research was preventive rather than therapeutic in nature. The subjects were expectant wives who had themselves gathered in groups of antenatal classes to prepare themselves for a new phase in their lives – motherhood.

The experimental intervention required no special extra resources, since it was conducted with the voluntary help of the patients' obstetricians and the hospital's public health nurses. Both the experimentals and controls received standard antenatal instructions as part of the regular program conducted by the public health nursing section of the hospital. We provided the experimentals with the special experimental instructional classes, while the controls continued to receive the same preparation that they and previous groups had been getting. The obstetricians and nurses contributed by rating the patients' postnatal emotional state on the simple five-step scale mentioned earlier. The ratings took place at the time of the patients' routine postnatal visits.

The reducing rehospitalization study also operated on a modest budget in comparison with the usual costs of treating discharged mental patients in community mental health centers. In 1981, it cost $1.54 per day per patient to pay patient peer leaders and part-time paraprofessional staff who served as resource persons.

Doing arithmetic analyses

Here again, you can design causal relation studies like these where you do not need complicated multivariate procedures. Chi-square with its simple arithmetic was used in both studies.

Table 7.2. *Main findings of the causal relation research on preventing postpartum emotional distress, presenting the mean number of changes reported by each of the experimental and control groups of mothers in antenatal classes and the percentage of each group judged as reacting normally in the postnatal period*

	N of Q_1 S's	Mean antenatal score	N of Q_2 S's	Mean change score	χ^2	p	N of S's judged	% of S's normal	χ^2	p
All experimentals (E)	73	4.5	62	1.6	11.8	<.001	85	85	9.8	<.01
All controls (C)	56	4.4	35	0.4			76	63		
Total	129		97				161			
C couples	27	4.6	14	0.1	16.0	<.001	38	66	7.3	<.01
E couples	44	4.8	38	2.0			54	89	2.0	N.S.
E wives	29	3.9	24	1.0	6.9	<.01	31	77	2.2	N.S.
C wives	29	4.2	21	0.7	0.4	N.S.	38	60		
Total	129		97				161			
All 1st half	66	4.3	41	0.7	4.9	<.05	79	70	1.9	N.S.
All 2nd half	63	4.4	56	1.4			82	79		
Total	129		97				161			
Normal S's	98	4.7	75	2.0	18.0	<.001	120	100		
Emotionally upset	31	4.7	22	−0.6			41	0	—	—
Total	129		97				161			

There was one degree of freedom for all of these calculations.

The experimental instructions of the research on preventing postpartum distress influenced the experimental expectant couples to make significantly more recommended changes than did the controls. Changes were reported in the follow-up postnatal questionnaires, which the women filled in while in the hospital maternity ward after delivering their infants. Patients who responded by making more recommended changes fared significantly better emotionally than did those who made fewer changes.

Tables 7.2 and 7.3 present some of the experimental data. Table 7.2 shows that experimentals as a group made an average number of 1.6 changes in the recommended direction, as compared with the controls' mean of 0.4 changes ($\chi^2 = 11.8$; $p < .001$). Only 15% of the experimentals responded with emotional distress to their maternity experience six weeks after delivery, as compared with 37% of the controls ($\chi^2 = 9.8$; $p < .01$). Six months postnatally, 2% of the experimentals (1 of 46) as compared with 28% of the controls (10 of 36) remained emotionally distraught ($\chi^2 = 9$; $p < .01$). As might be expected, women in the experimental group who attended classes for couples, where husbands attended with their wives, made the most recommended changes and experienced the least emotional distress.

The experimental groups of women in antenatal classes and their spouses made the following behavioral changes in their lives significantly more than did the control groups: (1) Wife increased her number of friends who were young wives; (2) wife decreased her emphasis on household tidiness; (3) wife obtained more help with the baby; (4) husband became more available to his wife and child; (5) wife continued outside activities but reduced them; (6) couple continued outside activities but reduced them; (7) couple arranged for a baby-sitter before delivery.

Table 7.3 presents two of these significant findings. The step the women took that affected their mental health most positively was to increase their social support groups to include more friends among couples with young children.

Tables 7.4 and 7.5 report additional research data. Note that there were changes in both a positive and a negative direction. For example, if a wife made more friends who had young children, her response was scored as a positive change; if a husband increased the number of nights he spent away from home each week and thus became less available to his wife, this was a negative change. Each woman received a positive or negative score based upon the net number of changes she and her husband made between the time she attended antenatal classes and delivery of her baby.

Researchers often use single numerical scores like these as measures of the overall effectiveness of a treatment program. This helps with data analysis, but it gives equal weight to each component in the final score.

Table 7.4 shows that the groups who were exposed to the largest amount of treatment (the *independent variable,* instructional information) were the most likely to respond by making the largest number of recommended changes (the *mediating variable*) (comparing independent and mediating variables, $\chi^2 = 15.1$; $C = .367$; $df = 4$; $p < .01$).

Table 7.5 shows that those groups who reported the largest number of recommended positive changes responded best emotionally (comparing

Table 7.3. *Selected mediating variable and dependent variable responses of subjects (behavioral responses reported by maternity patients = mediating variable; their associated postnatal emotional reactions = dependent variable)*

Response	Antenatal reported change		Comparing E's and C's		Postnatal emotional reaction		Comparing distressed and normal	
	E's N = 62 %	C's N = 35 %	$df = 1$ χ^2	p	Distressed N = 23 %	Normal N = 74 %	$df = 1$ χ^2	p
Made friends with young wives[a]								
More[a]	69.5	45.5	5.2	< .05	30	73	11.7	< .001
No more or fewer	30.5	54.5			70	27		
Stressed tidiness in the home[a]								
Less emphasis[a]	66	31.5	10.83	< .001	35	61	4.8	< .05
Same or more emphasis	34				65	39		

[a]Recommended change.

Table 7.4. *Frequency distribution of behavioral changes reported by subjects in various groups in antenatal classes. The independent variable (exposure to instruction) and the mediating variable (amount of behavior change) are compared by means of C, the contingency coefficient, and chi-square*

	1st & 2d half couples E groups	2d half wives E group	1st half wives E group	Both 2d half C groups	Both 1st half C groups	Total N of S's
Treatment group ranked by exposure to instructions						
Rank by amount of instruction	1	2	3	4	5	—
Subjects in group who reported changes						
Number of reported changes:						
+2 to +6	27	8	5	6	6	52
−5 to +1	10	4	8	13	10	45
Total	37	12	13	19	16	97
Percent who responded as instructed						
	73	67	38.5	31.5	37.5	—
Rank by amount of response						
	1	2	3	5	4	—

$C = .367$ ($C_{max} = .894$). $\chi^2 = 15.1$. $p < .01$. Larger percentages of women who made recommended changes in their lives came from the groups who received a greater amount of exposure to the content of the instructions.

the mediating and dependent variables for those who responded normally with those who were upset postnatally, $\chi^2 = 13.7$; $C = .35$; $df = 2$; $p < .001$) (R. E. Gordon, 1961).

Calculating chi-square and the contingency coefficient with small expected frequencies

In Table 7.5, 20% of the cells contained expected frequencies of less than 5. Tables 7.5A and 7.5B show how to calculate χ^2 and C when 20% or more of the cells contain expected frequencies of less than 5.

The data in Table 7.5 indicate that some antenatal women made a number of recommended positive lifestyle changes; others made no change or actually

Table 7.5. *Computing chi-square and C when many cells contain fewer than five members: frequency distribution of number of life changes reported by antenatal women and their subsequent postnatal emotional reactions*

	No. of behavioral changes reported[a]					Total N of S's
	< -2 & -2	-1 & 0	+1 & +2	+3 & +4	+5 & > +5	
Judged postnatal emotional ratings						
Normal[b]	1 (7.6)	19 (19.8)	19 (16.8)	27 (23.6)	8 (6.1)	74
Upset[b]	9 (2.4)	7 (6.2)	3 (5.2)	4 (7.4)	0 (1.9)	23
Total	10	26	22	31	8	97
Percentage rated *normal*	10	73	86	87	100	

Because the expected frequency is less than 5 in 20% or more (in 2 or 10 = 20%) of these cells, the 10 cells are collapsed into 6 cells, as shown below, before χ^2 is computed.

	No. of behavioral changes reported[a]			Total N of S's
	< -2 to 0	+1 to +2	> +2	
Judged postnatal emotional ratings				
Normal[b]	20 (27.5)	19 (16.8)	35 (29.7)	74
Upset[b]	16 (8.5)	3 (5.2)	4 (9.3)	23
				97

[a] Positive numbers represent behavioral changes made in the recommended direction; negative numbers, those made in the direction opposite to that provided in the instructions.
[b] Expected frequencies are shown in parentheses.
$\chi^2 = 13.7$. $df = 2$. $p < 0.1$. $C = .351$ ($C_{max} = .816$).

altered their lifestyles in a manner that might worsen their life situations. After delivery, the emotional reactions of all of these women were rated by experts as being either *normal* or *upset*.

Table 7.5 presents a frequency distribution of the numbers of postnatally rated *normal* women who made positive and negative lifestyle changes and gives the same data for postnatally rated *upset* women. The chi-square of 13.7 shows that there is a significant ($p < .001$) difference between these two groups in the numbers and direction of their antenatal lifestyle changes and in the postnatal ratings of their emotional reactions. We were thus able to reject the null hypothesis that there would be no significant difference between these two groups.

However, since we hypothesized that antenatal changes in different directions would produce different postnatal reactions in the two groups, we wanted to know if the large number of *normals* making positive changes might have accounted for the overall difference. This could mean that the negative changes (or lack of change) by the *upsets* had nothing to do with their postnatal ratings.

To determine whether or not lifestyle change was related to postnatal emotional reaction in each group (rather than in the group as a whole), we separated the groups according to their postnatal emotional ratings and applied a chi-square goodness-of-fit test to each. The rationale for doing so was that, if the lifestyle changes had nothing to do with the postnatal ratings, then the numbers of women making antenatal changes would be equally distributed across the range of possible changes for either groups or for both groups taken individually. This would mean that some other factor, unknown to us, could have been responsible for the differences between the two groups.

Determining goodness of fit

As always, the null hypothesis played devil's advocate and stated that our educated guess (that is, the research hypothesis) was untenable. But we had to make two null hypotheses, one for each goodness-of-fit test. These were: (1) Scores for antenatal lifestyle changes will be equally distributed across the range of changes for postnatally rated *normal* women, and (2) scores for antenantal lifestyle changes will be equally distributed across the range of changes for postnatally rated *upset* women.

Each of our null hypotheses postulates a distribution of lifestyle changes that, when plotted, forms a horizontal line on a graph. In each case, these points represent the expected values in the chi-square goodness-of-fit test. We shall work through the process for each group separately to exhibit the method. (In many studies, there would be only one set of expected values; in the research discussed here, there are two sets only because we are treating each group as a study in itself.)

For the postnatal *normal* group, the expected value at each point (if ratings for emotional reaction have nothing to do with number of positive antenatal changes) is the total number of *normal* women, 74 divided

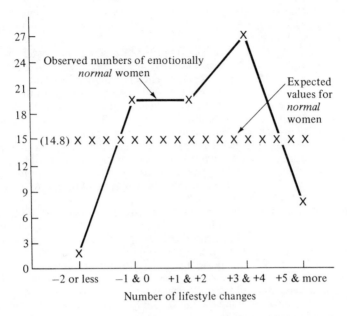

Figure 7.1. Curves comparing expected and actual numbers of women rated *normal* postnatally who made antenatal lifestyle changes.

by 5, the number of groups, or 14.8, that is, the number of *normal* women expected in each group as shown now:

Expected values for antenatal lifestyle changes: normals

No. of changes	< −2 & −2	−1 & 0	+1 & +2	+3 & +4	+5 & >+5
Expected number of women	14.8	14.8	14.8	14.8	14.8

The actual distribution of postnatally rated *normal* women was as follows:

Actual values for antenatal lifestyle changes: normals

No. of changes	<−2 & −2	−1 & 0	+1 & +2	+3 & +4	+5 & >+5
Observed no.	1	19	19	27	8

Figure 7.1 shows the two curves for the *normal* group: The flat horizontal line is produced by the expected values for the *normal* group; the line with the high scores for positive change shows the actual values for the *normal* group. The chi-square formula for a goodness-of-fit test is:

$$\text{chi-square} = \text{the sum of } (O - E)^2/E$$

where O = the actual score values and E = the expected score values.

Comparing the observed numbers of women with the expected values, we find that chi-square = 28.43, which confirms that the curve of obtained values is significantly different from the curve of expected values. The difference between the two curves is so large that there is a probability of only 1 in 1,000 ($df = 4$; $p < .001$) that the differences are due to chance.

Using the same procedure for the *upset* group, we find that the expected value for this group is 4.8 (23 *upset* women/5 groups = 4.6). (Although one could use Yates's correction here, there is no need to do so, since these are frequencies and the 4.8 could logically be rounded to 5. The result is essentially the same with or without the rounding.) In this case, the values are:

No. of changes	< -2 & -2	-1 & 0	$+1$ & $+2$	$+3$ & $+4$	$+5$ & $>+5$
Expected no.	4.6	4.6	4.6	4.6	4.6
Observed no.	9	7	3	4	0

The resulting chi-square is 10.69 ($df = 4$; $p < .05$), which indicates that the observed values are significantly different from the expected values. In other words, the two curves shown in Figure 7.2 are significantly different from each other.

However, note that the curve for *normals* was significantly different from the expected curve because there were high positive values (indicating that a large number of women made positive lifestyle changes); the figure for the *upset* women shows that the obtained values form a curve significantly different from the expected because a large number of women made zero or negative antenatal lifestyle changes. Thus comparing the curves for each group with a curve unaffected by postnatal ratings shows that each curve is different from the expected, but the curve for the *normal* women has large differences at the positive end of the scale, whereas the *upset* women show large differences from zero through the negative end of the scale.

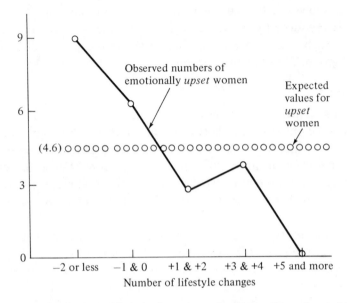

Figure 7.2. Curves comparing expected and actual numbers of women rated *upset* postnatally who made antenatal lifestyle changes.

A goodness-of-fit test, therefore, can exhibit the source of differences. This gives us more information than simply knowing that two groups are different from each other.

The study also considered whether *demographic characteristics* – education or socioeconomic position – made a difference. Upper- and middle-class and college-educated women responded significantly better to the instructions than did lower-class and less educated ones. As to background stresses, women with stresses in their past histories, such as death of a parent or severe personal illness, which are unrelated to social mobility, were significantly less likely to benefit from the special antenatal instructions.

A comparison of the characteristics of women who were distressed only at six weeks postpartum with those who remained distressed for six months showed that new wives with a history of illness and other problems were significantly more likely to recover emotionally after a short period of emotional distress. However, women who received less support in their new motherhood role from their husbands or relatives tended to remain distressed.

Dissemination and replication

If your research is successful and is part of a program supported by a state, agency, or corporation, you may be called upon to disseminate findings to sister agencies. If they and others can duplicate them, they will want to apply your treatments in their settings. Furthermore, a research finding is not automatically accepted until others have successfully replicated it in their settings.

Findings of the study on preventing postpartum distress were reported in presentations to local obstetricians and public health nurses, as well as in scientific and other publications. The new groups learned what information their antenatal patients needed and began to provide instructions themselves. Subsequently the postpartum reactions of 63 of their patients were evaluated. Only 11% of these women, to whom the nurses and obstetricians alone provided the special antenatal instructions, had undergone postpartum emotional distress. This compares favorably with 31% of the first 36 women in antenatal classes who received instructions in the experiment on preventing postpartum distress ($\chi^2 = 12$; $p < .001$). The latter group were those who received the least amount of information from other sources.

Follow-up studies

The benefits of psychiatric treatment are frequently impermanent. If you have developed a new successful procedure, you might wish to follow up your patients and review their status after they have left your care. A good time to look at them again is five years later.

Five years after completing the experiment above, we obtained follow-up information on 99 instructed women and 22 controls. The instructed women included both persons who had participated in the formal experiment and others who had received instructions from the obstetricians and public health nurses in the dissemination phase of the study. The instructed women were functioning significantly better than the controls five years after the conclusion of the experiment: 20% of the former were still experiencing emotional troubles, as compared with 46% of the controls ($\chi^2 = 6.9$; $p < .01$). The specially instructed women had subsequently given birth to significantly more children ($\chi^2 = 4.8$; $p < .05$) and had undergone fewer serious health problems, sex problems, or marital complications such as divorce or separation (R. E. Gordon, Kapostins & Gordon, 1965).

Dissemination of the research findings has been associated with a decline in incidence of emotional disorders of childbearing women (operationally defined as women aged 18–30 years who required psychiatric treatment for an emotional disorder during pregnancy or within six months after childbearing) from 6% (59 of 988 patients seen in private office practice) treated prior to reporting the program in the 1950s to less than 0.5% (1 of 210 patients) seen after its dissemination ($\chi^2 = 9.2$; $p < .01$). Because of our research and writing, our medical colleagues and others in the community considered us to be experts in the care of psychiatric maternity patients and sent these patients to us. Thus this decrease in incidence is impressive.

Additionally, analyses of social indicators revealed that infanticide in the state also declined in the same period from a mean rate of 4.9 per 100,000 before dissemination of the findings of the study on preventing postpartum emotional distress to 1.6 per 100,000 after the study was completed. In comparison, during the same periods the overall homicide rate in the state rose from a rate of 2.35 to 2.6 per 100,000.

The follow-up studies confirm the thesis that couples' making appropriate life changes during the wife's pregnancy and building good social supports help prevent emotional disorders of pregnancy and childbearing. The social indicator data provide support for the thesis.

This research led to modifications in the psychiatric care of couples with young children. The studies suggested the importance of counseling, educating, and training patients to make practical changes in their lives – reduce stresses, maintain a social life and other leisure-time pleasures, and, most important, build an environmental support network of helpful friends appropriate to the life situation.

In the investigation into reducing rehospitalization 10 months after discharge from the hospital 35% of the controls as compared with 17.5% of experimentals had required rehospitalization ($\chi^2 = 58.5$; $p < .0001$). The average total number of days of hospitalization for the CND patients was also much lower (7.0 days versus 24.6 days). Finally, significantly more CND patients functioned effectively without requiring any contact with the mental health system, inpatient or outpatient (52.5% versus 26%). CND members required far fewer hours of outpatient psychiatric care (201 versus 1,158; $p < .01$).

The patients' Likert scale responses indicated that those who took leadership responsibilities in the CND did not feel their roles were stressful. They indicated that their job was a positive, growth-producing experience for them. As a result of this finding, CND now tries to increase member participation in middle-management leadership.

Critique of examples

A study like the research on preventing postpartum distress benefits from having an easily defined, time-limited, measurable endpoint – delivery – and a measured period following it. Further, the women could be followed through their physicians. On the other hand, the main data-collection phase of the study on preventing postpartum distress occurred in the late 1950s, before the advent of objective, standardized scales for measuring emotional disorder. Thus, the research suffers from methodological flaws that need not occur today. Too, the physician and nurse raters might not have been blind as to which subjects were experimentals and which controls. (They were not informed, but with a little questioning of their patients they could have figured this out if they wished.)

Researchers must deal with these realistic problems all the time. Even if good standardized tests had been available in the 1950s to rate the postpartum women's emotional responses six weeks, six months, and five years after delivery, would the 45 obstetricians have spent their time filling in the sheets? Most likely not. Someone would have had to visit over 500 patients' homes on three separate occasions to administer the standardized tests. This kind of effort is what costs big money in research – probably more than $15,000 in this instance.

Like the study on preventing postpartum distress, the reducing rehospitalization research also suffers from some methodological flaws. Except for the single assessment of the importance of leadership, this study did not measure and evaluate the effects of CND's various mediating variables – the contribution of training in peer counseling, in providing mutual support, in leisure activities, and the rest. Thus the relative importance of each of these steps cannot be weighed in the same manner as can the changes made by the new wives shown in Table 7.4.

To follow up on the mediating variables was a far more complicated and expensive task with the experimental and control patients in this reducing rehospitalization study than it was in the research on preventing postpartum emotional distress. In the latter study it was easy to collect mediating variable data by noting when the patients, both experimentals and controls, expected to deliver. Then they filled in the follow-up questionnaire in the hospital ward where they resided after giving birth to their babies.

On the other hand, the patients in the reducing rehospitalization study, like the geriatric psychiatric patients of the psychoeducational treatment research and the veterans of the geographic unitization study, had all been discharged from the psychiatric hospital and were living throughout the community in their own residences. The reducing rehospitalization experimentals did gather once a week at the CND meeting where they could be interviewed. That is how the peer leaders filled in the Likert scales. But the controls could only be reached by letter, telephone, or visits to their homes. As mentioned in connection with the research on preventing postpartum distress, making home visits is an expensive, time-consuming process. (To call on the veterans in the geographic unitization research cost $10,000.) Further, many patients had moved without leaving forwarding addresses. These considerations explain why it is best to conduct controlled studies in settings where the patients naturally gather – classes, wards, aftercare clinics, and so on – where you will not need to track them down as the experiment progresses.

Findings from the causal relation studies reported here have been fed back into patients' therapeutic programs, thus completing loops in the continuing spiral of assessment, evaluation, and research leading to improved quality of therapy. The same process has been applied with other groups.

Some needs assessment studies of college students were followed up by controlled experiments with 432 college students. In response to psychoeducational instructions in a college orientation program for freshmen, the experimental group took significantly more of each of the following steps than a matched group of controls: (1) They conferred more with faculty and student advisers about their plans and college work. (2) They planned their programs of courses more effectively. (3) They were more likely to drop courses if they discovered themselves over their heads in them. (4) They avoided overloading themselves with outside jobs or extra courses for which they were not well qualified. (5) They prepared themselves in advance for difficult courses. (6) They took extra reading and English courses if their test results indicated they needed them. (7) They chose friends who were doing well in school and steered clear of those who got into trouble with academic authorities. (8) They spent more of their spare time on the college campus. (9) They did not hurry to finish college, but proceeded at a comfortable pace.

As a result, the experimentals did significantly better in the following areas: (1) They made a better mean grade-point average. (2) They were less likely to be placed on academic probation. (3) They were more likely to make a B average or better. (4) They made fewer trips to the college health office. (4) They were less likely to require disciplinary action for campus misbehavior. (5) They were less likely to quit college or to be asked to leave for academic or other reasons. These studies have been published in journal articles and a book (R. E. Gordon & Gordon, 1963: 296–9).

Using the microcomputer

Good software programs are now available to perform both simple and complicated parametric and nonparametric statistics on microcomputers. We encourage you to obtain an office or home computer and the necessary software. Statistical analysis and graphing programs for the Macintosh computer and the IBM-PC and related personal computers are easy to use.

Most practicing clinician-researchers can get along fine with a microcomputer to do their statistics. You can handle moderately large sets of data and compute most statistical tests, simple statistics, multivariates, and nonparametrics with one. Only when you are pressed for time or are conducting many studies with large masses of data involving thousands of cases do you need a mainframe computer setup.

Publishing

Because obstetricians and their patients are especially interested in preventing postpartum emotional distress, findings from the studies on this subject appeared first in the obstetric literature. Later they were incorporated in a book for the layman (R. E. Gordon & Gordon, 1960; R. E. Gordon, Gordon & Gunther, 1961). They provided experimental evidence of the value of psychoeducational treatment and mutual support in preventive psychiatry. They also led to the use of these techniques in psychiatric office and hospital practice. Subsequently, the psychiatric, sociological, obstetrical, and psychological literature has cited the findings (Gartner & Riessman, 1982; Hopkins, Marcus & Campbell, 1984; J. H. Williams, 1974). The literature for women has repeatedly reported the 11 instructions for expectant mothers (Boston Women's Health Book Collective, 1973; Cogan, 1980).

The Community Network Development (CND) program of the research on reducing rehospitalization, like the observed relation geriatric psychoeducational program, has been approved by government officials for implementation in outpatient mental health settings in several states' public mental health systems. This peer-managed social support system for chronic mental patients is also being cited in the psychiatric and sociological literature. These studies contribute scientific evidence that supports the efforts of the self-help and mutual-help group movements. The repeated observation that helpful environmental supports improve the functioning of psychiatric patients and other groups has led to the general acceptance of a psychiatric law: *Supports boost functioning* (Gartner & Riessman, 1982).

Publishers who are familiar with your other studies in a series are likely to be receptive to new reports that confirm, negate, or clarify earlier investigations. Find a challenging research theme and pursue it. Not only will publishers welcome your contributions; your patients will also gain from your efforts.

Summary

This chapter has shown how to conduct experimental causal relation research. It has considered both preventive studies and therapeutic ones aimed at improving patients' functioning. It has emphasized a continuing process of clinical assessment, monitoring, evaluation, and research leading to improved patient care.

The chapter also discussed when and how to use a consultant in statistics or experimental design, and mentioned some statistical programs for the microcomputer.

8. Developing a theory: the functional level equation

A theory is the highest stage in the spiral of research that begins and ends with generation of a hypothesis. We have examined the functional level concept and followed its development through earlier research stages: hypothesis, measurement, and observed relations. This chapter discusses a theory that states that functional level is positively correlated with coping skills, directive power, and environmental supports, and that it is inversely correlated with aggravating stress and biomedical impairment. This theory can be expressed in an equation, the *functional level equation.* This chapter will show how the theory was generated and is being tested.

Definition

A theory provides a description or operational definition of how to (1) classify, (2) predict, or (3) control events. It is based on measurement, observed relation, and causal relation researches. A theory's principal characteristic is that it summarizes the results of several researches and attempts to make generalizations based on their findings. A theoretical article integrates research findings and need not present original data. It stimulates new hypotheses that need to be tested.

To be of any scientific value, a theory must be stated in terms that allow it to be tested. For example, Harvey's theory of the circulation of the blood was of no use in those countries where dissection of the human cadaver was not allowed. Tests on other mammals would not have verified Harvey's theory, since suggesting a relationship between humans and animals would have violated current religious beliefs. If the social and legal climate had not changed to make verification of his theory acceptable, it would have remained in the realm of idle speculation. On the other hand, phrenology, the theory that propounded character analysis by an examination of cranial protuberances, was impossible to test

172

because repeated excursions into the living brain merely for the purpose of checking out one's character would have been required. Unlike the circulation of the blood, personality characteristics disappear when the organism dies. Hence these would have had to be checked out and confirmed in vivo, which procedure could hardly be justified; nor would there have been many volunteer subjects available for such experimentation. Idle speculation has its place in helping to generate more concrete ideas, but it is only well-formulated, testable theory that can result in contributions to the scientific knowledge in a field like psychiatry.

This chapter briefly reviews studies mentioned previously to show how a single functional level theory, related in part to the APA's *Diagnostic and Statistical Manual (DSM-III)* (1980), can account for the findings reported. It presents the factors in relation to one another as an equation, and reports on new studies designed to test how well the equation succeeds in classifying the phenomena reported. Finally, it shows whether the theory can predict and control events and can stimulate research.

A new theory – the ABCs of psychiatry

In the early 1980s George Albee (1982) began to publish a series of reports on preventing psychopathology and promoting human potential that presented the following formula:

Incidence = (Stress + Organic factors)/(Coping skill + Self-respect + Support)

He hypothesized that emotional disorders could be reduced or prevented by efforts to decrease the problems in the numerator of the equation – stress and organic factors – and to increase those in the denominator – coping skill, self-respect, and support. This simple but elegant formulation is appealing because it seems to wrap up all the measurable variables important in psychiatric treatment and prevention in one equation containing only six biopsychosocial elements. Despite the infinite variability of individual patients, and indeed all persons, there are only a finite number of measurable factors that are important in mental health and disease. Can there be only six crucial variables?

Many psychiatric tests and scales attempt to measure the important variables in psychiatric treatment. But most objective tests and scales, including those shown in chapter 4, are limited in scope. When taken together, they can be very helpful in the care of patients, as is shown in Table 4.1 and in the modular psychoeducational treatment programs mentioned in chapter 6. But to administer enough scales to accomplish all the benefits shown in Table 4.1 for each patient in a clinical treatment program would take an unreasonable amount of time and effort. Could Albee's formula be adapted to help in quantifying psychiatric treatment?

Later Gartner and Reissman published an article on self-help and mental health (1982). In it they cited both Albee's formula and the studies on preventing postpartum emotional distress and on reducing rehospitalization of chronic mental patients described in chapter 7. Their report stimulated us to reexamine what the study on preventing postpartum distress had shown from the perspective of Albee's prevention formula.

The experimental treatment had:

1. Reduced the aggravating stresses affecting the antenatal women – an element in the numerator of Albee's formula (e.g., wife decreased her emphasis on household tidiness)
2. Decreased their biomedical problems as a resultant dependent variable – another numerator element (e.g., fewer wives suffered postnatal emotional distress)
3. Increased their leisure-time coping skills – a denominator element in the Albee formula (e.g., wife and couple both continued outside activities but reduced them; couple arranged for a baby-sitter before delivery)
4. Increased their environmental supports – another denominator element (e.g., wife increased her number of friends who were young mothers and obtained more help with the baby; husband became more available)

The research made no effort to measure the patients' self-respect, the third element in the denominator of Albee's formula. But women with better educations and higher socioeconomic positions, who held greater power and control over resources, responded better than did those with a poorer education and lower socioeconomic status, who held less directive power. The overall outcome of the research effort was to reduce the *incidence* of emotional distress among the experimental groups as compared with the controls. Furthermore, five-year follow-up studies showed that, after wide dissemination of the findings of the preventive research, incidence of maternity psychiatric disorders and of infanticide declined significantly in the area (see chapter 7).

The reexamination of the psychiatric maternity research seemed to support Albee's equation. His formula, with slight modification, might not only be used in classifying the variables involved in preventing psychiatric problems, but might also serve to describe what quantitative changes take place during psychiatric treatment. *DSM-III* could be used to quantify part of the formula.

We modified the Albee formula in five ways in order to use it as an equation for measuring the psychiatric treatment process:

1. The fraction was inverted to its reciprocal
2. The names of its elements were changed to improve their mnemonic qualities
3. The term "directive power" replaced "self-respect"
4. The formula incorporated Axes I through V from *DSM-III*
5. The new theory was expressed as an equation that showed the relationship between the interacting predictor variables in the fraction and the dependent variable – current functional level, as shown here (R. E. Gordon & Gordon, 1985):

$$\text{Functional level} = f\frac{\text{Coping skill} + \text{Directive power} + \text{Environmental support}}{\text{Aggravating stress} + \text{Biomedical impairment}}$$

or $FL = f(C + D + E)/(A + B)$, where f means "function of." Rating scales have been selected or developed for measuring each element of this equation. (Each scale ranges from 1 to 7; thus neither the denominator of the fraction nor the numerator can ever go to zero.) *DSM-III*'s Axis IV aggravating stress scale and Axis V premorbid functional level scale appeared previously in chapter 2. Scales B through E for measuring the remaining variables appear in Tables 8.1 to 8.4.

In the new theory, self-respect is not considered a separate variable because the work with modular psychoeducational treatment had shown that it was a coping skill that could be trained. One of the modules taught in the program discussed in chapter 6 successfully helped patients build their self-esteem (see Table 6.1). On the other hand, directive power, the control over human and material resources, is highly important in psychiatry and in life. People with a higher socioeconomic position, a better education, and more control and direction over human and material resources are less likely to develop psychiatric disorders. Furthermore, they respond better to preventive and therapeutic efforts.

In the equation, *functional level* (*FL*) considers quality of life in social relations, in work and school, in performance of activities of daily living, and in management of stress and physical impairments. Well-functioning, mentally healthy people maintain their high performance despite aggravating stresses (*A*) and biomedical impairments (*B*) – adversities that may overwhelm their less-adjusted fellows – because of the strength of their coping skills (*C*), directive power (*D*), and environmental supports (*E*). *FL* is placed at the core of comprehensive psychiatric treatment and rehabilitation. The *FL* score provides a single numerical measure that can be used to assess a patient or a group of patients and to measure response to therapy.

The theory leads to a hypothesis that comprehensive, successful psychiatric treatment should help patients to raise their *FL* scores. After they finish therapy, they should function at a higher level than they ever did before. A test of this hypothesis will be discussed later.

Both therapeutic and preventive psychiatry help patients to improve some or all of their coping skills, directive power, and environmental supports, and to decrease or manage their aggravating stresses and biomedical impairments, as shown above with antenatal women.

FL is measured globally on instruments such as the Axis V scale of *DSM-III*, or by computing it from a modified *FL* equation, which will be discussed below. (Recently, *DSM-III-R* introduced a new nine-step scale for functional level.)

Aggravating stress (*A*) is related to ongoing realistic problems. Many standardized instruments like the well-known Holmes and Rahe (1967) scale, as well as the maternity questionnaire and the Axis IV scale of *DSM-III*, have been developed to measure the severity of stressors. The Axis IV scale is currently used to measure *A* in the studies discussed below.

Biomedical impairments (*B*) include the diagnoses described in the first three axes of *DSM-III*, severity of illness, factors associated with genetic vulnerability, early sensitization, aging, obesity, malnutrition, substance abuse and other behavioral excesses, lack of exercise, and apathy. Medical, surgical, psychopharmaceutical, and behavioral treatments affect the *B* variables. Researches on coronary artery and other psychosomatic diseases, and on college students' blood chemical responses to stress, reported previously, dealt in large part with relationships between aggravating stresses and biomedical impairments. Current studies with brain imaging techniques, with neurotransmitters and receptors, and on the genetics of neuropsychiatric disorders are all investigating the biomedical impairment variable. They may lead to the development of standardized tests that help measure components of *B*.

The biomedical impairment scale currently used, shown in Table 8.1, is based on the level of medical or nursing care patients need, their depen-

Table 8.1. *The biomedical impairment scale currently being studied*

1. Superior Health: (1) No illnesses; (2) Eats a proper diet and maintains normal weight; (3) Exercises regularly; (4) Sleeps well; (5) Does not abuse any substances; (6) Needs no health care from professionals.
2. Good Health: May have a disease or test abnormality which is controlled by self-medication, diet, or exercise; Needs professional health care only to monitor self-care (includes psychodynamic and behavior therapies, use of oral psychotropics, self-managed diabetes, peritoneal dialysis).
3. Fair Health: Has an illness which requires regular medical management such as injected medicines and blood tests (prolixin, lithium, blood sugar); is able to live outside an institution.
4. Mildly Ill: Needs open ward care in a crisis stabilization or short-term treatment unit, or partial hospitalization because behavior, symptoms, or treatments are not manageable in the home (includes hemodialysis); Needs minimal health care from staff.
5. Moderately Ill: Requires hospital care in a locked psychiatric ward because behavior represents a threat to self or others; needs a full complement of health care staff.
6. Seriously Ill: Requires hospital care in a locked ward with special checks (at least every 15 minutes) for suicide threats, recovery room care after electroconvulsive therapy or surgery.
7. Critically Ill: Requires constant one-to-one suicidal watch or supervised care in a seclusion room, restraints, an intensive care unit, or an operating room.

dency, and their dangerousness. It employs a step system similar to those used in many child/adolescent or behavioral inpatient treatment programs.

Progress in reducing biomedical impairments among outpatients who are functioning at the lower, healthier levels of the *B* scale may be more precisely measured by any of the numerous instruments for assessing depression, anxiety, and other symptoms (see chapter 4).

Many acute medical and surgical patients with uncomplicated physical diseases, e.g. pneumonia or appendicitis, return to a high level of functioning when they recover from their biomedical impairments. However, many persons with chronic physical diseases – hypertension, limb amputation, paraplegia, renal disease, diabetes, and so forth – as well as many with psychiatric disorders, are not so fortunate. The latter may never have attained a high functional level. Thus, unlike many surgeons and internists, psychiatrists (and physicians in rehabilitation medicine) cannot content themselves with just treating and assessing the *B* variable.

Coping skills (*C*) are learned throughout life. Dynamic psychotherapy

Table 8.2. *The coping strengths and deficits scale currently being studied*

7. Superior: (1) Person has very effective personal/social skills – communicates and asserts self well (CA), is neither too passive nor too aggressive; (2) Solves personal problems and conflicts, and provides leadership appropriate to role in life (PSL); (3) Has effective academic/vocational skills (AV) – studies effectively and performs appropriately in class or on the job (has no examination phobias or stage fright), obtains and keeps jobs, does not take on more than can handle well, gets along well with fellow students or employees, teachers or supervisors, and subordinates; (4) Enjoys leisure (L) – plays and relaxes well; (5) Builds and maintains self-esteem successfully and controls emotional impulsivity, anxiety, and depression (SEC); (6) Sets reasonable long- and short-term goals (G) and pursues them successfully; (7) Performs basic living (BL) skills well – maintains a clean living area and good personal hygiene (PH), manages personal budget and finances well (Bu), transports self satisfactorily either by driving a car or using public transportation (T), eats a proper diet (Di), and manages medications satisfactorily (M).

   Patients may receive a score 1, $\frac{1}{2}$, or 0 on each of the seven elements of the Coping (C) Scale. In the case of the Basic Living (BL) subscale, performance of only one of the five elements receives a rating of 0, performance of 2–3 is rated $\frac{1}{2}$, and of 4–5 is rated 1. Patients who have acquired a Coping Skill, but lost it temporarily because of their illness, receive partial credit for the ability.
6. Very Good: Score of six of above.
5. Good: Score of five of above.
4. Fair: Score of four of above.
3. Poor: Score of three of above.
2. Very Poor: Score of two of above.
1. Grossly Impaired Coping Ability: Performs none or one of above.

teaches them, as does modular psychoeducational treatment (see Table 6.1). People cope with inner thoughts, painful feelings, their own and others' aggressions, and difficult external situations. The *C* scale (Table 8.2) measures both strengths and defects and also points out to treatment personnel which areas of an individual's functioning to assess and treat.

Directive power (*D*) is related to socioeconomic status: educational, vocational, and financial position – "clout." Persons with high *D* control important environmental reinforcers: other people and material resources. As discussed in chapter 6, psychiatric treatment can lead to improved directive power. *D* is measured on a scale (Table 8.3) that has been adapted from the well-known instrument of Hollingshead and Redlich (1958).

Environmental support (*E*) systems include the patient's family and friends. The studies of maternity patients, college students, and chronic

Table 8.3. *The directive power scale currently being studied*

This scale combines four factors – occupation, formal education, residence, and continuing education – into one measure. It uses the same seven occupational positions as did Hollingshead and Redlich (1958) in their Index of Social Position, but in reverse order: 7. Executives and proprietors of large concerns and major professionals; 6. Managers and proprietors of medium-sized businesses and lesser professionals; 5. Administrative personnel of large concerns, owners of small independent businesses, and semi-professionals; 4. Owners of little businesses, clerical and sales workers, and technicians; 3. Skilled workers; 2. Semi-skilled workers; and 1. Unskilled workers.

It closely follows their educational scale, again with the order reversed: 7. Graduate professional training with receipt of a graduate degree; 6. Standard 4-year college or university graduation; 5. Community college graduation; 4. Started college but did not earn a degree; 3. High school graduation; 2. Completed junior high school (ninth grade); 1. Less than a ninth-grade education.

Residence is ranked on a scale which ranges as follows: 7. The most exclusive neighborhoods; 6. Middle-class single-family neighborhoods; 5. White-collar-worker neighborhoods; 4. Blue-collar neighborhoods; 3. Public low-cost housing; 2. Rooms and apartments in inner city or factory districts; 1. The poorest tenements in slum neighborhoods.

The mean of the scores on these three subscales is obtained. If the patient is enrolled in and pursuing an accredited program of courses and is completing each segment as required for a degree, a union, a licensing board, or a profession, etc., each of the three scores is raised one full level to give the final average D Score.

Full-time students are ranked according to their parents' home and occupational level and their own educational attainment. Since they are attending school, their mean score is raised one level. Full-time housewives receive the occupational rank of their husbands. Divorced and separated persons are rated as if they were single, with consideration to any alimony and other allowances they receive. Retired persons receive ratings according to their incomes from their pensions and other resources, their occupations in part-time or other jobs or professions, and their attendance in continuing education classes, just the same as if they were not retired.

mental patients all point to the importance of E supports in preventing or treating emotional and mental problems. Edmunson and her colleagues reported on the benefits to patients of positive feelings toward the environmental network and reciprocally warm relationships with fellow network members, and the disadvantages of negative feelings and irritations (see chapter 7). These findings, and those of Tolsdorf (1976) and Pattison (1977) on size and other characteristics of psychiatric patients' and normals' social networks, provided the items for measuring E. Like its counterpart for measuring coping skills, the E scale (Table 8.4),

Table 8.4. *The environmental supports and problems scale currently being studied*

© 1983 R. & K. Gordon

7. Superior: (1) Network contains at least 20 persons; (2) Majority are not kin; (3) Not more than one-half of persons in network know each other; (4) Most relationships are helpful, warm, and friendly; few are destructive, troublesome, or irritating; (5) Most relationships are reciprocal, although there are some relationships with persons both above and below the patient; (6) There are no key linking members without whom the network would fall apart; (7) There are both close and distant relationships.
6. Very Good: Network contains 15–19 persons and five of the characteristics above; most relationships are warm and helpful.
5. Good: Network contains 12–14 persons and four of the characteristics above; most relationships are warm and helpful.
4. Fair: Network contains 10–11 persons and three of the above.
3. Poor: Network contains 8–9 persons and two of the above.
2. Very Poor: Network contains 6 or 7 persons and one of the above.
1. Grossly Impaired: Network contains 5 or fewer persons and none of the above.

---

reminds the treatment team what important areas of patients' support systems to consider in preparing their treatment plans.

Assessing reliability and validity of the *FL* equation and its scales

The reliabilities of the Axes IV and V scales have been tested and reported in *DSM-III*. We reexamined the reliability and validity of these scales and the others of the *FL* equation in a pilot study that used 20 descriptive case histories taken from 10 long-term patients' psychiatric records. Each patient had undergone both inpatient and outpatient treatment. Initially, two of eight experienced mental health professionals – six psychiatrists, one psychiatric nurse, and one psychiatric social worker – scored each patient's current *FL* using both the Axis V scale and all five *A, B, C, D,* and *E* scales. A first case history described the patients on entering treatment; a second portrayed the patients after they had undergone considerable therapy. The mental health professionals obtained coefficients of reliability ranging from .83 to .86 for all six scales and the computed *FL*-equation values.

The same case histories were subsequently presented to approximately 200 experienced mental health professionals in four group sessions. Their mean group scores were correlated with the mean score obtained by each pair of the initial eight mental health professionals. The correlations were in the .82–.87 range.

Validity was determined by correlating the eight professionals' ratings of current functional level on the Axis V global scale with scores computed with the five scales in the *FL* equation. Each professional rated the *A* (stress) through *E* (support) scales on five of the psychiatric patient case histories, and current Axis V globally on a different five. No one scored the same patient case history in both manners. The coefficient of validity between the current *FL* score computed with Scale *F* above (the Axis V scale) and functional level computed by the formula $FL = f(C + D + E)/(A + B)$ was .86 ($p < .01$).

Graphically, the relationship between computed raw *FL* values and Axis V ratings was curvilinear. However, the square roots of raw scores produced a straight-line relationship with Axis V scores. A least squares analysis produced the following equation, which provides the best-fitting straight line for converting raw *FL*-equation data into *DSM-III* Axis V scores:

$$FL = 7.8 - 2.1 \sqrt{(C + D + E)/(A + B)}$$

The procedures above for fitting a curve to data, analyzing the shape of a curve, transforming a curve, and using the least squares method are beyond the scope of this book. Persons who wish to pursue this topic further should consult Horst's *Psychological Measurement and Prediction* (1966).

There are independent measures of Scale *A*'s (Axis IV's) and Scale *F*'s (Axis V's) reliability in *DSM-III*, and of the reliability and validity of Scale *D* in Hollingshead and Redlich's book (1958). But the assessments of the reliability and validity of the *B*, *C*, and *E* scales and of the equation as a whole need to be replicated in other full-scale research settings, and with patients in clinical treatment, not just with sample case histories taken from patients' records. Further, the accuracy of ratings by newly trained and inexperienced personnel needs to be studied. Such studies are being conducted.

Correlational studies are also needed between *FL*-equation scores and those with other psychiatric tests and rating scales, such as those mentioned in chapter 4. No one of the latter rating scales assesses all six elements of the equation, but some go into greater detail than do the equation's scales.

As new data become available from continuing clinical studies testing the uses of the *FL* equation, some of the scales, the multiplier, and other

relationships in the equation, as well as the validity and reliability correlations can be expected to be refined. However, the equation's measures
are all ordinal scales, and it is clinically useful in its present form.

Classification

A theory must be able to classify phenomena to which it relates. Therefore, when you develop a new theory or study one proposed by someone
else, examine how well it classifies information in its field. With respect
to the functional level equation, look first at some of the studies and other
information reported earlier in this book, and examine whether it can
classify:

1. Objective factors measured in psychiatric tests
2. Objective outcome measures of psychiatric researches
3. Patient goals in psychiatric treatment
4. Staff roles of psychiatric treatment team members
5. Program goals of psychiatric treatment facilities
6. Amount of patients' distress

Classifying objective factors with psychiatric tests

Numerous rating scales and tests are available for psychiatric treatment
staff to measure patients' problems and their progress in therapy. Many
of these were discussed in chapters 4 through 7 as well as elsewhere in
this book. Inspecting Table 4.1, you can see that all the scales measure
one or more of the six A through FL elements of the FL equation. However, all these instruments are narrower in scope than the FL equation;
none address the entire range of A through FL problems and patients'
progress in resolving them to the same extent as do the equation and its
scales. It might be possible to put together a battery of tests that might
cover all the functions described in Table 4.1, and thus those potentially
served by the FL equation, but it would take a great amount of staff time
to administer it. Moreover, the equation alone provides all the benefits
of the psychiatric rating scales listed in Table 4.1.

Classifying therapeutic studies

The section "A New Theory" earlier in this chapter showed how the six
elements measured by the FL equation corresponded to the objective cri-

teria used in measuring the outcome of the studies on preventing post-partum emotional distress. What about the other researches reviewed in this book?

Look back at another study and consider what objective measures were used to assess the needs and progress of patients. The combined treatment researches (see chapter 6) assessed such objective measures and indicants of patients' response to treatment as their (1) moving into a new home or community – measures of aggravating stresses; (2) needing hospitalization, rehospitalization, or electroconvulsive therapy – measures of biomedical impairment; (3) returning to work, school, or college – measures of directive power; and (4) continuing or terminating marriage – measures of environmental supports. Thus the research studies were examining four of the elements of the patients' functional level equation.

Classifying goals of psychiatric treatment

Review of Meldman, McFarland, and Johnson's comprehensive *Problem-Oriented Psychiatric Index* (1976) and examination of over a thousand psychiatric patients' records in 26 different hospital settings – public and private, state, university, federal, nonprofit, and for-profit – confirmed that goals and objectives of patients' treatment plans could be classified in one or other of the six A through FL categories of the FL equation. A list of frequently observed goals and objectives and their categories is shown in Table 8.5 (R. E. Gordon & Gordon, 1983).

Classifying professional staff assignments

An early description of the FL equation in a paper on professional roles in psychiatry noted that the elements of the equation reflect the major assessment and treatment roles of the members of the psychiatric treatment team. However, well-trained psychiatrists alone can assess and treat every variable in the equation.

The primary therapist, often the psychiatrist, is largely responsible for assessing and treating aggravating stresses. Only psychiatrists understand fully the physiological, biochemical, anatomical, and pathological aspects of the biomedical impairments component. In most states, only they can hospitalize or medicate a psychiatric patient. Thus they are the primary assessors and therapists of the biomedical impairment variable. Nurses, behavioral psychologists, occupational and activities therapists, and other staff supplement their efforts.

Table 8.5. *Classification of goals of psychiatric treatment (data from a review of 50 psychiatric case records from 26 psychiatric hospitals)*

Aggravating stress (A)
Reduce stress
Deal with conflict areas
Ventilate feelings about problems

Biomedical impairment (B)
Control inappropriate behavior
Decrease delusions
Decrease hallucinations
Increase reality testing
Keep patient out of trouble
Control nervousness and anxiety
Elevate mood
Decrease depression
Control compulsions and obsessions
Reduce tensions
Decrease violent behavior
Decrease religious preoccupation
Decrease crawling on knees
Reduce weight
Increase weight
Abstain from alcohol
End abuse of drugs
Begin to exercise
Improve sleeping pattern

Directive power (D)
Address financial problems
Discuss disability issues
Return to work
Repair disorganized lifestyle and
    inability to hold a job
Return to school
Perform volunteer work

Environmental support (E)
Improve communication with parents
Replace separated wife and family
Support dependency needs
Improve family feedback
Improve relations with family
Decrease antisocial behavior

Coping skills (C)
Basic living (*BL*)
    Learn to budget
    Improve personal hygiene
    Improve appearance
    Use public transportation
Communication/Assertion (*CA*)
    Control impulsive behavior
    Overcome loneliness
    Decrease dependence
    Develop normal voice tone
    Increase range of affect
    Control anger
    Increase assertiveness
    Increase compliance
    Improve trust
    Decrease competitiveness
    Improve interpersonal relations
    Decrease aggressive behavior
    Control problems with authority
    Decrease maladaptive attention
        seeking
    Overcome shyness
    Increase independence
Set goals/Clarify values (*G*)
    Establish a better value system
    Improve long-term goals
Leisure (*L*)
    Learn to enjoy leisure
Academic/Vocational (*AV*)
    Improve attendance in class
    Learn to find jobs
Problem solving/Leading (*PSL*)
    Decrease jealousy
    Decrease sexual confusion
Self-respect/Emotional control (*SEC*)
    Increase self-esteem
    Improve self-control

Occupational and other activities therapists are particularly involved in assessing and treating coping skills and deficits; they are assisted by psychotherapists. Educators and vocational trainers are best qualified to assess and enhance the directive power variable. Social workers are primarily responsible for assessing and improving patients' environmental supports. The team as a whole works to improve patients' *FL*.

Classifying treatment programs and facilities

Rating the patient's scores on the *FL* equation, obtaining the *strain ratio,* and calculating the predicted amount of treatment required helps therapists to determine what type of treatment setting is most appropriate for the patient. Thus the equation and theory also meet this test.

With many patients, treatment to raise patients' functional levels often addresses the elements of the equation in alphabetical order. In the first phase of treatment, patients may be acutely ill – depressed, agitated, hallucinating, possibly a danger to themselves or others, and severely dysfunctional. Acutely ill hospitalized patients generally need *crisis intervention* first to reduce aggravating stresses, and medications and other therapies to decrease abnormal symptoms, feelings, and behavior (biomedical impairments).

Once the extreme manifestations of patients' psychiatric illnesses have come under control and they are more amenable to therapy, they can receive training in improving their coping skills. Those with poorer premorbid functional levels (*pFL*) – with low *C* scores and high strain ratios (*SR*s) (1.2 or above) – may require further treatment in *specialized inpatient or day-hospital programs,* in treatment settings where there are good skills-building occupational and other therapy programs available.

Higher-functioning patients with fewer coping-skill defects receive follow-up care in an *outpatient setting* where psychiatrists, other primary therapists, and rehabilitation personnel can exert a major influence in helping them acquire a variety of useful social and other coping skills. There is little point in enrolling patients in formal schooling when they cut most of their classes, ignore their homework, and pay little attention when they get into class. This is a major problem with seriously disturbed children and adolescents, which helps account for why many need *long-term inpatient* treatment. They must first improve these and other academic coping skills. Likewise, placing seriously ill adult patients in competitive jobs can be a waste of time and effort unless they have first learned the coping skills necessary for getting to work on time, bathing regularly, dressing properly, and avoiding arguments and fights with their bosses and fellow workers.

Educators and vocational therapists perform the assessments and treatments related to patients' educational, vocational, and other attainments that give them direction and control over their lives and resources – their directive power. With seriously impaired patients with low FLs, efforts to improve patients' educational and socioeconomic status (their D) must follow preeducational and prevocational coping-skill training. Therefore, D programs usually require a specialized, *long-term hospital or day-hospital* setting for more chronically ill patients.

Poorly functioning patients with low FL scores and high SRs who are residing in state institutions and in *long-term private, tertiary care hospitals,* which often are located 50 or more miles away from their homes, cannot do much to raise their environmental support levels while they remain in full-time hospital residence. Sessions in the hospital may help patients to improve their family relations and their ability to make and keep friends, and to increase their other coping skills – communicating, asserting, and leading. But the main job of improving their social networks must occur in *community-based programs* like the Community Network Development (see chapter 7) when they return to their home community.

These examples all show that the functional level equation and theory serve well to classify psychiatric rating scales, outcome measures of psychiatric researches, patient goals in psychiatric treatment, psychiatric staff roles, and types of treatment facilities.

Prediction

A theory must be able to predict events. According to the functional level theory, the elements of the FL equation should predict (1) psychiatric patients' treatment needs, (2) amount of distress in a community, and (3) functional progress in treatment. Furthermore, research that makes predictions (hypotheses) about the effects of a new treatment should control for the possible effects of extraneous variables. The FL equation identifies extraneous variables that are not always controlled; these may account for why some research studies fail to support their research hypotheses.

Predicting psychiatric patients' treatment needs

Higher scores for coping skills, directive power, and environmental support in the numerator of the equation – the wellness variables – are associated with patients' better functioning. Larger scores for aggravating stress and biomedical impairment in the denominator – the sickness variables – contribute to worse functioning. Psychiatric treatment is associated with efforts to improve wellness and to decrease sickness. The *FL* equation predicts that psychiatric patients with higher scores for aggravating stress and biomedical impairment will require longer periods of treatment, as measured by length of inpatient hospital stay (*LOS*) or numbers of outpatient sessions; those with better premorbid functional level (*pFL*) scores will require less treatment. The formula

$$LOS = f(A + B)/pFL$$

expresses this relationship, where *f* means "function of."

A series of researches examined the validity of the hypothesis contained in this expression. First they looked at the correlations of aggravating stress (the Axis IV score of *DSM-III*), *pFL* (the modified Axis V score), and their ratio, A/pFL, which was called the strain ratio (*SR*), with *LOS* [SR = Axis IV score/(8 − Axis V score)]. Data from some of these studies were presented in Table 4.4 (R. E. Gordon, Jardiolin & Gordon, 1985; G. R. Zanni, personal communication, 1986).

Table 8.6 presents data from 150 inpatients and outpatients. It shows that *LOS* and amount of outpatient treatment are related to *SR*. *SR* appears to be an index of patients' vulnerability to stress. Higher Axis IV (*A*) scores seem to be more important among outpatients – in the greater number of treatment sessions they received – while poorer *pFL* was especially related to inpatients' longer *LOS* (R. E. Gordon & Gordon, 1987).

The *SR* and the *FL* theory from which it developed can explain the observation that some people – chronically ill mental patients, in particular – often appear to relapse without any apparent stress, while others seem to bear enormous burdens of aggravating stress without collapsing. Consider for example a chronic schizophrenic man with an Axis V premorbid functional level score of 6, *very poor functioning,* and thus a transformed functional level score of (8 − 6 =) 2. As long as he is subjected to no stress, his Axis IV score is 1, and his strain ratio = 1/2 = 0.5. He probably will be able to live outside a mental hospital, perhaps in a halfway house. But let him get into a serious argument with his roommate, a mild stress scored in *DSM-III*'s Axis IV at the 3 level, and his strain ratio then becomes 3/2 = 1.5. Now he may need a period of hospital care. On the other hand, a working woman with many friends, who has performed well at difficult jobs with occasional feelings of tension,

Table 8.6. *Predicting psychiatric inpatients' and outpatients' treatment needs with their scores on Axis IV and Axis V scales and their strain ratios*

	Outpatient sessions			Inpatient days in hospital			
	1–5	6–20	21+	<30	30–59	60–89	90+
No. treatments							
Mean Axis IV score	3.60	3.85	3.80	3.83	3.95	3.89	3.88
Mean converted							
Axis V score[a]	4.93	4.53	3.92	4.28	4.09	3.78	3.38
Strain ratio (SR)	0.73	0.85	0.97	0.90	0.97	1.03	1.25
Number of patients	22	44	27	18	22	9	8

Notes: Outpatients, $N = 93$; inpatients, $N = 57$; total $N = 150$.

For outpatients and inpatients together, correlations between amount of treatment and strain ratio: Spearman's rho = .94; $p < .01$. Between amount of treatment and Axis IV scores: rho = .79; $p < .05$. Between amount of treatment and Axis V scores: rho = $-.89$; $p < .01$.

Note the overlap between *SR*s of outpatients who came for 21 or more treatment sessions and of inpatients who stayed in the hospital for fewer than 29 days. This phenomenon is related to the fact that some patients' insurance policies provided better coverage for inpatient than for outpatient coverage.

[a]Converted Axis V scores are obtained by subtracting the raw score from the number 8.

has performed well at difficult jobs with occasional feelings of tension, has a premorbid functional level score of 3, *good functioning* in *DSM-III*'s Axis V, and thus a functional level of $(8 - 3 =) 5$. For her to need hospital care, she most likely would have to undergo a severe aggravating stress such as a marital separation, a major financial loss, or a serious physical illness (*A* score of 5 in *DSM-III*). Any of these would send her strain ratio up to $5/5 = 1$. Many patients with a strain ratio of 1 require inpatient psychiatric care (R. E. Gordon, Jardiolin & Gordon, 1985).

The studies examined next the influence of the biomedical impairment variable – psychiatric patient diagnoses on Axes I and II of DSM-III and the severity or stage of the illnesses. As discussed in chapter 5, multiple regression (R) equations that included all five of *DSM-III*'s diagnostic axes, *SR*, and stage (severity) of illness (along with patient age and sex) accounted for between 41% and 62% of the variance in psychiatric patients' *LOS*. Patients with certain diagnoses like schizophrenia and those with more severe illnesses remained longer in treatment; those with other disorders, such as adjustment reaction, required less treatment (Gordon, Vijay, et al., 1985). These researches confirmed that the functional level equation and theory, and the strain ratio derived from it, predict amount of treatment psychiatric patients receive and their treatment needs.

Predicting amount of distress in a community

Chapter 5 presented data from a study that hypothesized that *SR*s of patients in faster-growing, more stressful communities would be higher than those in slower-growing ones. This theme is related to findings about social mobility and distress mentioned previously. Table 5.1 in chapter 5 presents the data from this research. In each setting the mean *SR*s of outpatients in the fast-growing counties (1.3 and 1.2) were much higher than those of outpatients in the slower-growing one (0.9). The *FL* equation explains the difference in *SR*s between patients in faster- and slower-growing communities.

The studies also showed that the 51% of child patients in the rapidly growing communities came from homes where they had a single parent, usually a divorced mother. Looked at from the perspective of the *FL* equation, this observation can be interpreted as follows: The child patients' *FL*s decreased as a result of increased aggravating stress related to moving to a stressful community, decreased directive power associated with declining socioeconomic status related to their parents' divorce, and fewer environmental supports associated with separating from the family and friends they left behind.

Other predictions

We are testing the hypothesis that strain ratio scores are correlated with the decision by the Social Security Administration to provide benefits to psychiatrically disabled workers. We also hypothesize that strain ratio scores will predict acts of aggression in violence-prone patients. When stress increases, especially stress related to aggravating relationships with friends and relatives (see chapter 7), or functional level decreases, and thus the strain ratio rises, the tendency to violence to self or others should increase.

Assessing patients' progress in treatment

The theory considers functional level as a variable affected by the interaction of the five components in the fractional part of the *FL* equation.

Table 8.7. *Comparing functional outcome and symptomatic outcome of outpatient psychiatric treatment*

Session frequency	Outcome of treatment (%)			No. of patients
	Worsened	No change	Improved	
41+				*14*
Functional	0	55.5	44.5	
Symptomatic	0	14.5	85.7	
21–40				*18*
Functional	10.5	55	34.5	
Symptomatic	0	11	89	
11–20				*33*
Functional	5	62.5	32.5	
Symptomatic	6	24	70	
6–10				*35*
Functional	12.0	64.0	24	
Symptomatic	0	20	80	
1–5				*132*
Functional	14.5	77.0	8.5	
Symptomatic	2.5	61.5	36	
Total no. of patients				232

These differences are statistically significant. For symptomatic change, $\chi^2 = 41.8$; 2 *df*; $p < .0001$. For functional change, $\chi^2 = 30$; 4 *df*; $p < .001$.

The equation and theory suggest that comprehensive psychiatric treatment should affect the whole person – sometimes all six elements of the equation. Therefore the theory predicts that measurements of improvements in patients' functional level (*FL*) after psychotherapy should differ from those of their symptomatic (*B*) improvements.

Table 8.7 compares findings from a group of 232 patients assessed for symptomatic and for functional response to treatment (R. E. Gordon, Gordon, Plutzky, et al., in press). The Axis V scale was used as a measure of current functional level. The table shows that functional improvement was not nearly as large as symptomatic improvement. Clinical experience with patients suggests that functional measures of patient progress are probably more useful than symptomatic ones, since they are probably better related to long-term improvement and recidivism. This too is a researchable question stimulated by the use of the equation.

The data show that by using the two different kinds of measures of patient progress, clinicians and researchers obtain more information than they would if they used only symptom change. Patients required fewer treatment sessions to improve symptomatically than they needed to improve their level of functioning. Program evaluators might well assess patients both symptomatically and functionally, and use the information for quality assurance purposes – peer and utilization reviews, for instance.

These findings show that, as predicted, the equation's functional level and biomedical impairment elements measure different entities; in a full evaluation of a patient's response to treatment, the change in *FL* is probably the most important in psychiatry.

Performing research

The observations above may also apply to research studies, particularly those that evaluate the effectiveness of new medications. This kind of research often uses instruments that assess patients' response along a single dimension – depression or another symptom. But many patients with a psychiatric disorder, unlike those with appendicitis or lobar pneumonia, are usually suffering from more than just painful symptoms; they usually are also enduring handicaps related to deficits in their coping skills and social supports. These handicaps reduce their functional levels and render them vulnerable to relapses when subjected to new aggravating stresses after they have recovered from the acute phase of their disorders.

This is particularly true with patients with a history of substance abuse or violence. They may respond well symptomatically to treatment in the controlled social structure of the hospital. But then they return to a possibly aversive and unsupportive environmental support system in the community. There new symptoms of their disorder are provoked. Research on the effects of various treatments or on predicting future behavior of discharged patients would do well to consider all the elements of the *FL* equation, not just the *B* variable.

Matching experimentals and controls in research

Chapter 2 and several subsequent chapters emphasized the importance of random selection of patient samples for research. With the use of random sampling or matched experimental and control groups, individual differences among patients/subjects do not confound the results of the research.

Most good studies, particularly those concerned with the therapeutic effects of new psychotropic medications, attempt to match experimentals and controls on age, sex, and *DSM-III*'s Axes, I, II, and III, which relate to the biomedical impairment variable. Then they can state that the responses of the experimental group that are significantly different than those of the controls are not due to extraneous variables. In performing the matching, researchers usually consider demographic factors, some of which may involve the patients' socioeconomic and educational status (features of directive power) and marital status (related to environmental supports). But few investigators pay systematic attention to the aggravating-stress, coping-skill, and other environmental-support elements of the *FL* equation. Unfortunately, few even consider matching on Axis IV and Axis V of *DSM-III* and on severity of illness.

Therefore, many research studies produce unpredicted, contradictory findings. These probably are related in part to the fact that patients of the same age, sex, marital status, and socioeconomic status, and with the same Axes I, II, and III psychiatric diagnoses, still may differ from each other. They may have better or worse *A*, *C*, and *E* factors in their lives that affect their overall functioning (*FL*) and their response to experimental interventions. However, if patients were carefully matched on all six elements of the equation, including diagnosis and severity of illness, as well as on age, sex, marital status, and other demographic variables, they should be less likely to differ in their response to new methods of treatment. This hypothesis, which stems from the functional level theory, can readily be tested in the conduct of new research studies.

Control

Theories suggest ways to control events. The *FL* equation indicates that changes in any of the five predictor variables in the equation's fraction should affect functional level. And changes in *FL* should be accompanied by one or more changes in the five variables in the fraction. Therefore systematic efforts to improve any or all of patients' coping skills, directive power, and environmental supports in therapy, combined with plans to reduce or control aggravating stress and biomedical impairments, should produce higher *FL*s and improvements in patients' mental health. The goals of psychiatric treatment, as shown in Table 8.5 and in the book by Meldman and his associates (1976), are these.

This section shows how the equation can be used in planning and controlling a patient's treatment and in measuring his or her progress in therapy. Furthermore, systematic collection of a number of patients' scores on each variable in the equation provides data for monitoring patient care, evaluating patient programs, reviewing resource utilization, upgrading quality of care, and planning research – all efforts at systematically controlling psychiatric events.

In the following psychiatric case history, the goals and objectives of a patient's psychiatric treatment plan and her progress in therapy are analyzed in terms of the *FL* equation. The patient's treatment shows how controlling the predictor variables in the equation results in changes in the outcome variable – the patient's functional level.

Planning and quantifying treatment

The case history of Marna that follows illustrates the use of all six variables in the equation to quantify various components of a patient's psychiatric treatment. (To preserve confidentiality, the true identity of the patient and others mentioned in this section has been disguised.) The five predictor scales are used to obtain an initial assessment, to help plan the therapeutic process, and to measure progress. Marna's case is not intended to be a model of patient care. It provides only the information needed for diagnosing her illnesses, scoring the equation's scales, developing her master treatment plan, and monitoring her progress in therapy (Alderman, Gordon, Gordon, Ahsanuddin & Slaymaker, 1984).

However, the use of the *FL* treatment approach favorably affects the treatment process, especially when contrasted to the use of traditional treatment planning. Currently, in developing and updating the comprehensive treatment plan the therapist(s) (1) must determine what are each patient's problem areas – there is no systematic way to cover every aspect of the patient's difficulties, and important areas may be left out; (2) must devise ways of assessing the problems objectively; (3) cannot pool data and compare progress from groups of patients, since they have not been assessed with the same measures; (4) is often bored, since the process is tedious and may take a considerable amount of staff time.

In contrast, the *FL* equation approach (1) points directly and systematically to the six (*A* through *FL*) areas where the patient needs to make improvements; (2) objectively assesses each of these areas before treatment on the same six scales; (3) helps the patient and the therapist(s) to develop objective treatment plans quickly; (4) makes the process enjoyable to both staff and patient, especially since they can readily understand the importance of treating each of the six areas addressed; (5) measures progress quantitatively in each of the six areas, as an intrinsic part of the therapeutic process; (6) can pool and compare group data for each of the six scales on which the patients have been assessed.

Marna's case history now illustrates the *FL* approach to treatment planning.

Illustrative case history – Marna

The first psychiatric hospitalization of this 40-year-old divorced mother of four children aged 4–18 began when she attempted suicide by overdosing on Tofranil. After her local general hospital had treated the acute symptoms of the drug overdose she was transferred to the referral hospital and treated on the inpatient psychiatric unit for depression. The patient had received outpatient treatment at her local community mental health center for depression related to problems in managing her children and conflicts with her divorced third husband. Her two previous husbands had also divorced her. The events which precipitated her overdose were the loss of her job as a beautician, the unexpected death of her boyfriend in an automobile accident, and the death of her second ex-husband, who fathered one of her children and provided some support for the child. Her Master Treatment Plan follows:

MASTER TREATMENT PLAN FOR ADULT PATIENTS
Functional Level Approach
© R. & K. Gordon 1983, 1984

Instructions
   Number problems in each category consecutively. Set measurable long-term (LTG) and short-term (STG) goals and expected time for completion. Name person responsible for carrying out different treatment modalities and their frequency.

A – Aggravating Stresses
Problem Descriptions and Assessments
   List stresses and rate them using Aggravating Stress Scale (1,4).

Scores	Problem Number
	A1. Marna has recently lost an ex-husband as well as her boyfriend with whom she lived and upon whom she was very dependent for emotional support. Her two oldest children are leaving home to enter college.
	A2. Her third ex-husband is resisting her demands that he provide more assistance in the care of their four children and greater financial and emotional support for her.
	A3. The beauty shop where she worked has gone out of business and she is unemployed.

Scores	Problem Number

A: 5
Severe Stress

B – Biomedical Impairment
Problem Descriptions and Assessments
　List impairments and rate them using the Biomedical Impairment Scale.

B1. The patient requires treatment on a locked ward with supervision to prevent suicide.

B2. Marna's grief over the death of her live-in boyfriend remains unresolved.

B3. She feels guilty and fearful about what others will think of her for attempting suicide and requiring treatment in a psychiatric hospital.

B4. Patient has multiple somatic complaints – headaches, anhedonia, insomnia, anorexia, memory deficits, and increased irritability which precede the onset of her menstrual period.

B: 5
Moderately Ill

C – Coping Skills
Problem Descriptions and Assessments
　List skills and rate them using Coping Skills Scale.

Basic Living (BL)

Personal Hygiene and Orderliness (Pho)
Marna is neat and tidy in appearance and keeps her living area on the ward clean and orderly.

Pho: +

C1. Managing Meals and Diet (Di)
She cooks well, but eats sparingly, and not a balanced diet.

Di: 0

Budgeting (Bu)
She manages her small budget satisfactorily.

Bu: +

Transportation (T)
She owns and drives a car wherever she needs.

T: +

C2. Medication Management (M)
She manages her medications poorly, and had overdosed on her psychotropic medications.

M: 0

BL: 1/2

C3. Communicating and Asserting (CA)
Marna is demanding and manipulative in relating to others. She initiates conversations

Scores	Problem Number
	C3 *(cont.)* readily, but maintains a self-centered perspective. She is unable to recognize and appreciate other people's points of view. She lacks insight into these deficits.
CA: 0	
	C4. Problem-Solving and Leading (PSL) She has little ability to cope with major problems in her life. Her only present leadership role is that with her children, but they largely go their own ways with little effective direction or control from her. She attempted once to own her own beauty shop but failed because of her lack of leadership ability with her employees as well as her poor bookkeeping and record keeping skills.
PSL: 0	
	Vocational/Academic Skills (VA) Marna works hard and has never had any trouble in getting or keeping a job. As a child she went to school regularly, did not miss classes, and was not tardy.
VA: 1	
	Leisure (L) **C5.** She enjoys dancing, playing cards, and going on outings with her younger children. Since the death of her boyfriend she cannot participate in the first two activities.
L: $\frac{1}{2}$	
	Self-Esteem and Emotional Control (SEC) **C6.** At the time of the illness the patient feels worthless. She is overwhelmed by the losses she has suffered. Her self-image has always depended upon the attitude of others, her parents as a child, her men as an adult. She is fearful about what people will think of her now that she is in a psychiatric hospital and has attempted suicide. She was upset upon turning 40 at her last birthday and the loss of her youth.
SEC: 0	
	Setting Goals (G) The patient's primary goal in life is to find a man upon whom she can lean and depend.
G: 0	

Total C: 2
Very Poor

D – Directive Power
Strengths and Problems
   Describe and score the patient's Directive Power (D) in terms of the D Scale.

D1. Home (Ho)
Prior to her illness Marna lived with her boyfriend and her four children in the large

Scores	Problem Number
Ho: 5	**D1** (*cont.*) house she owned in a lower-middle-class neighborhood in a city located 200 miles from the referral hospital. Her blood relatives live in Georgia, more than 500 miles from her home in Florida.
Ec: 3.5	**D2. Economic (Ec)** She had worked steadily as a beautician until one month prior to admission when her employer went out of business. On one occasion she tried to run her own shop, but gave it up because personality clashes led to her employees' repeatedly quitting. She also found keeping up with paperwork, bookkeeping, and tax forms very difficult, burdensome, and time-consuming.
Ed: 3	**D3. Education (Ed)** She completed only one year of high school prior to attending and completing a one-year course in cosmetology.
Ce: No	**D4. Continuing Education (Ce)** She has not pursued any further studies.

Average D: 4
Fair

E – Environmental Supports (E)
Strengths and Problems
   Describe and score the patient's environmental supports in terms of the E Scale.

Size: 10	**E1. Network Size (Size)** Network contains only ten persons. Marna's four children, her parents, sister, and brother in Georgia, a former husband with whom she has infrequent, but largely negative contacts, and one fellow beautician with whom she had worked. She experiences considerable stress in being a single parent with four children.
Kin: 0	**E2. Percentage of Kin (Kin)** Nine of the ten members are kin.
Know: 0	**Percentage of Network Who Know Each Other (Know)** All nine of her kin know each other.
	E3. Helpfulness (Help) Her relationships with her parents and siblings are helpful, but distant. Relationships with her ex-husband aggravate

Scores	Problem Number
	E3 (*cont.*) her, and those with her children strain her, since she cannot manage them alone and
Help: 1/2	cannot lean on them.
	E4. Reciprocity (Rec) She tries to depend on others, particularly
Rec. 0	her men, and cannot reciprocate fully.
	Close and Distant Members (C/D)
C/D: 1	There are both close and distant members.
	E5. Key Members (Key) Her dead boyfriend was key to more than half of her support system. His loss was a
Key = 0	major factor in precipitating her illness.

TOTAL E: 3
Grossly Impaired

INTERVENTIONS A – **Aggravating Stress Interventions**
Problems

Short & Long Term Goals	Treatment and Time for Attainment	Responsible Person & Frequency of Contact
A1. Loss of loved ones – two oldest children, live-in boyfriend, and ex-husband		
STG: Obtain assistance from her unmarried sister to manage home, care for younger children, and provide emotional support	Involve sister; 1 week	Social Worker (SW) & Sister; as needed
LTG: Learn to cope with losses	Individual Therapy; 2 months	Individual Therapist (IT), t.i.wk
A2. Conflict with ex-husband		
STG: Clarify nature, extent, and reasonableness of her demands. She and ex-husband will understand each other's individual styles and expectations	Family Therapy; 3 weeks	SW; once/wk

Problems

Short & Long Term Goals	Treatment and Time for Attainment	Responsible Person & Frequency of Contact
LTG: Determine patterns of marital conflict which led to repeated divorce	Individual Therapy; 2 months	Individual Therapy; t.i.wk
LTG: Assist patient and her ex-husband to negotiate new acceptable arrangements	Train negotiation skills Individual Therapy and Open Group; 3 months	IT and Occupational Therapist (OT); t.i.wk

A3. Loss of job and financial stress

STG: Obtain unemployment insurance	Assist patient to apply; 2 weeks	SW; as needed
LTG: Prepare to obtain job when she leaves hospital. Consider owning own business	Vocational Testing & Counseling; 2 months	Vocational Rehabilitation (VR); once/wk
LTG: Explore other sources of economic security	Inventory patient's assets and potential sources of income. Investigate boyfriend's and ex-husband's life insurance	SW; as needed

Overall measured A Goal:

STG: Reduce patient's A level from 5 to 3; 2 weeks		
LTG: Continue patient's A level at 3; 2 months		

B – Biomedical Impairments Interventions

B1. Attempted suicide

STG: Prevent suicide	Locked Ward and suicidal precautions Antidepressant medications	M.D. & Nursing Staff; as needed

Problems

Short & Long Term Goals	Treatment and Time for Attainment	Responsible Person & Frequency of Contact
B1 (*cont.*)		
LTG: End suicidal behavior	Cognitive Therapy for depression	IT; t.i.wk
	End ward restrictions; 3 weeks	M.D. & Nursing Staff

B2. Unresolved grief over sudden death of boyfriend

STG: Develop understanding of normal grief process	Individual Counseling; 2 months	IT & Chaplain; once/wk
LTG: Work through grieving process	Individual Counseling; 2 months	

B3. Guilt over suicide attempt & fear of others' attitudes

STG: Develop insight and evaluate reality of guilt and fear	Evaluate and clarify goals and values Individual Therapy	IT; t.i.wk
LTG: Learn to test and cope with reactions of others	Group Therapy; 2 months	Dynamic Group Therapist; t.i.wk

B4. Multiple somatic symptoms preceding her menstrual period

STG: Evaluate the duration and severity of symptoms and their relation to her menstruation	Observe and chart patient's behavior and reports of symptoms; 1 month	Nursing staff; as needed
LTG: R/O Premenstrual Syndrome or other organic etiologies	Gynecology consult; in 4 weeks Testing for biological causes Premenstrual medications	Gynecologist, M.D. & Lab
LTG: Divert self-centered attention. Gross motor activity to improve general circulation and normalize neurotransmitters	Recreational ward activities to involve patient in exercise and pleasurable activity	Recreational Therapist (RT); daily
	Relaxation training	AT; t.i.wk

Problems

Short & Long Term Goals	Treatment and Time for Attainment	Responsible Person & Frequency of Contact
Overall measured B Goals:		
STG: Reduce B level from 5 to 4; three weeks LTG: Reduce B level from 5 to 2; three months		
C – Coping Skill Interventions		
C1. Poor dietary management		
STG: Become aware of poor dietary habits and how she can change	Provide balanced meals. Group Nutrition and Meal Planning sessions; three weeks Continue eating proper diet; three months	Dietician; t.i.wk
C2. Poor medication management		
LTG: Learn the proper use of medications	Group Medication Sessions; three weeks	RN; t.i.wk
C3. Interpersonal skill deficits in communicating and asserting. Manipulative style, self-centered perspective, lack of insight, and inability to recognize other people's point of view		
STG: Become aware of her dependent and manipulative styles in communicating and asserting. Explore how these problems affected her past relationships. Get feedback on the effects of her behavior and interactions	Individual Therapy, open Group and Milieu Therapy Staff provide feedback to patient when she displays these characteristics; two weeks Individual and Open Group Therapies	IT, GT, RNs RNs IT; t.i.wk
LTG: Learn more effective communicating and asserting skills. Model new behavior after others who are more skilled than she	Encourage observation of other skills	GT; t.i.wk RNs

Problems

Short & Long Term Goals	Treatment and Time for Attainment	Responsible Person & Frequency of Contact
C4. Difficulty in solving personal problems and in leading others, in being the head of a single-parent household with four children		
STG: Clarify what stresses are occurring in present home situation	Individual Therapy; two weeks Family Therapy; two weeks	IT; t.i.wk SW once/wk
LTG: Learn effective problem solving and leadership skills. Apply them to avoid and relieve stresses in the home. Learn to apply above skills to managing others outside the family	Individual and open Group Therapy; two months Training in problem solving; decision making	IT, OT; t.i.wk
C5. Deficient leisure skills		
STG: Explore interests and potential for developing new leisure skills	Recreational skill testing; one week	RT
LTG: Develop new leisure skills. Attend offered leisure activities when restrictions end	Recreational Therapy; two months	RT OT; once/wk
C6. Defective self-esteem and poor emotional control		
STG: Discuss loss of self-image as result of deaths of boyfriend and ex-husband. Explore what losses mean to her	Individual Therapy; two weeks Individual Therapy	IT; t.i.wk
LTG: Learn to control anxiety, depression, and excessive grief, and to accept loss	Cognitive Therapy for anxiety, depression; two months	IT, OT; t.i.wk
C7. Inability to set either short-term or long-term goals		
STG: Develop insight into how her lack of goals contributed to her depression and sense of worthlessness	Individual Therapy; two weeks	IT; t.i.wk

Problems

Short & Long Term Goals	Treatment and Time for Attainment	Responsible Person & Frequency of Contact
LTG: Learn to set short-term and long-term goals	Open Group Therapy; Goal setting training; three months	OT; t.i.wk

Overall measured Coping Skill goals:

STG: Raise C level from 2 to 4 in three weeks		
LTG: Raise C level to 6 in three months		

D – Directive Power Interventions

D1. Distance of her home from her relatives

STG: Explore possibility of her moving to Georgia to live closer to her family	Family Therapy; two months	SW; once/wk
LTG: If she decides to move, find therapist in Georgia	SW; in two months	SW; once/wk

D2. Inability to manage own business due in part to lack of formal and continuing education

STG: Explore her motivation and capability for managing her own beauty shop	Vocational Testing and Counseling; two months	Rehabilitation Therapist
LTG: Improve her English, writing, mathematics, and bookkeeping skills in General Education Diploma (GED) classes	GED classes; 3 months; continue after discharge	Patient Educator

Overall measured Directive Power goal:

Raise patient's D level from 4 to 5 in three months		

E – Environmental Support Interventions
Problems

E1, E2, and E5. Poverty of social network and predominance of kin

STG: Improve her contacts with fellow patients	Assign her a roommate as soon as possible – 2 or 3 days	RN
	Encourage socialization with other patients	RN, RT, IT
LTG: Develop the skills required to establish a wider circle of friends and improve her support system	Individual Therapy; two months	IT; t.i.wk
	Women's Open Group; two months Local Single Parents Support Group in the community. Transfer to home branch after discharge; three months	SW; as soon as possible

E3 and E4. One-sided, aggravating relationships with ex-husband and others

STG: Patient, ex-husband, and children learn to recognize their problems with and express their grievances to each other	Family Therapy with patient and family together and separately; two weeks	SW; once/wk
	Open parenting group	OT; t.i.wk
LTG: Family Support and Negotiation Training for all older family members	Family Therapy; three months Open Group Negotiation Training; two months	SW; once/wk OT; t.i.wk

Overall measured Environmental Supports goal:

Raise patient's E level score from 3 to 4 in two months

The patient's diagnostic formulation was as follows:

Axis I: Major depressive episode.

Axis II: Personality disorder with mixed features.

Axis III: Premenstrual syndrome.

Axis IV (A – Stress) score: 5 – *severe stress* – death of boyfriend and second husband; loss of employment; difficulties with third husband; and two eldest children leaving home.

Axis V score: 4 – *fair* – fair premorbid functioning (pFL: 4). Did reasonably well at work and in managing and supporting four children.

Strain ratio ($SR = A/pFL$): 5/4 = 1.25.

Current functional level (cFL): 2 – *very poor* current functioning. (Note that this score is equivalent to a score of 6 on the Axis V scale.)

Estimated length of hospitalization: 90+ days (See Table 8.6).

Measuring therapeutic progress

The paragraphs that follow continue the description of Marna's progress in therapy. They illustrate how progress can be quantified.

By the time of her first treatment-plan update in the sixth week of her hospital stay, Marna's current FL had been raised to 3. She had achieved many of the short-term goals of her treatment plan. Her sister had come down from Georgia to manage her household and care for her younger children while she was in the hospital. This helped reduce her Axis IV score (A – stress) from 5 to 4. Her new SR (A/pFL) of 4/4 = 1 indicated that she was making satisfactory progress in treatment. After 10 weeks of treatment, Marna was discharged from the hospital. In less time than most patients with her initial SR, she had accomplished all the goals of her comprehensive treatment plan. Medications and medication training for both her psychiatric and premenstrual disorders had reduced her B (impairment) score from 5 to 2. The social worker's helping Marna arrange to receive unemployment benefits, plus insurance from both her deceased boyfriend's and ex-husband's life insurance policies, had helped her further reduce her A (stresses) score from 5 to 3.

Her psychotherapy and skills training sessions gave her insight into her personality problems as well as the resources to change. She improved her self-reliance and her skills in communicating, asserting, problem solving, leading, using leisure, relaxing, and managing guilt, anxiety, and depression. Her C (skills) score rose from 2 to 7. Family therapy dealing with providing mutual support and negotiating helped prepare her for managing family problems effectively and for making more and better friends. General Education Diploma (GED) classes, which continued after her discharge from the hospital, were also preparing her to run her own business, if she wished. Her directive-power (D) level consequently rose from 4 to 5.

Marna and her family all agreed that everyone would be better off if she and her two younger children moved back to Georgia with her relatives while her two older children went off to college. During trial visits with her family in Georgia before her final discharge from the hospital, Marna signed up to continue her GED classes at night school there and joined a local chapter of a single parents' support group. In both she could associate with groups of men and women coping with concerns and interests similar to hers, and with whom she could expand her circle of dependable friends. Her E score rose from 3 to 4 as a result.

Proceeds from the sale of her house in Florida provided her with additional financial security and the funds to open her own business if she desired. After leaving the hospital she lived with her parents in Georgia; thus her daily living costs were less than they had been in Florida. She easily obtained a job as a beautician soon after moving to Georgia. She also contacted a psychiatrist there with whom she continued her treatment as an outpatient. The doctor made sure that she continued to follow a proper diet as well as supervising the use of her psychotropic and other medications.

By the time Marna left the hospital, her current FL score had returned to its premorbid level of 4 *(fair functioning* in *DSM-III* terms), and her A (stress) score remained at 3 *(mild stress)*. Her SR of $3/4 = 0.75$ is like that of other patients receiving brief outpatient psychiatric treatment shown in Table 8.2. However, like others who are benefiting functionally from outpatient psychiatric care, she continued to come for treatment.

In her aftercare, she continued GED classes until she mastered the academic skills needed in business and passed the examinations in the other subjects required to receive her diploma. Her psychiatrist continued her medications and treated her with both individual and group psychotherapy every week. She continued to raise her E (supports) score by making friends in her new neighborhood, increasing the size of her social network, and improving the quality of the relationships – the helpfulness, reciprocity, and percentage of nonkin members. Gradually her E (supports) score rose to 7, the highest level. As she settled into her new home and job, her A (stress) score decreased from 3 to 1.

In less than nine months from the time she entered therapy, Marna had greatly improved her level of psychosocial functioning, increasing her current FL from 2 (and premorbid functional level from 4) on admission to the hospital to 5 – *good functioning* (3 on the Axis V scale). Her Axis IV score had declined from 5 *(severe stress)* to 1 *(no aggravating stresses)*. Her SR of $1/5 = 0.2$ was like that of normal persons who do not need any psychiatric treatment.

Summarizing, Marna's scores on entering treatment were:

$$A = 5; B = 5; C = 2; D = 4; E = 3;$$
$$cFl = 2; \text{Axis V score} = 5; \text{and } SR = 1.25$$

After 10 weeks of treatment, upon leaving the hospital, her scores had changed to:

$$A = 4; B = 2; C = 7; D = 5; E = 4;$$
$$cFL = 4; \text{Axis V score} = 4; \text{and } SR = 0.75$$

The numerator scores in her FL equation rose from 9 to 16, while those in the denominator decreased from 10 to 6. Her current functional level, as measured by Axis V, was 4. Half a year later, Marna's scores were:

$$A = 1; B = 2; C = 7; D = 5; E = 7; \text{Axis V score} = 3; SR = 0.2$$

Now her numerator scores totaled 19 and her denominator ones, 3. Now her current Axis V scale score was 3.

Evaluating the individual patient's progress in treatment

Once norms have been established with a large number of people on a test such as the MMPI, Stanford – Binet intelligence test, or Axis V scale, you can find out how individual patients compare with others on the instrument, and how much progress they have made.

Researchers are beginning to obtain normative data with the Axis V scale. For example, the data in Table 4.4 show that the standard deviation for 77 psychiatric patients was 1.0, and for another 149 was .97. If data from thousands of patients continue to show that the SD of the Axis V scale is about 1.0, then a change from an Axis V score of 6 to one of 4, such as was described in Marna's case above, would represent an improvement of two standard deviations. The further change to an Axis V score of 3 would represent an improvement of three standard deviations.

Planning treatment with the aid of a personal computer

We are seeking to develop a computer-aided treatment plan for use with personal computers. It would help therapists to assess the components of the *FL* equation by means of its six rating scales in the same systematic manner as they were measured in Marna's case history. The computer program measures premorbid functional level with the Axis V scale and calculates the strain ratio (*SR*). With data on diagnosis, severity of illness, sex, and age, it prints out a description of the patient and his or her strengths and weaknesses, computes the expected length of treatment, suggests short-term and long-term goals in treatment, and develops a possible treatment plan. Members of the treatment team modify the plan to suit their own and their facility's programs. Table 8.8 shows an excerpt from a treatment plan that uses this computer-aided approach.

Upgrading quality of care

The functional level equation and theory contribute to controlling the quality of care of patients. Feedback from evaluating programs, monitoring patient care, and reviewing utilization by means of the equation and its elements can lead to improved patient treatment. Scores from each of the *A* (stress) through *E* (supports) scales and from the *FL* equation as a whole can be pooled and analyzed statistically.

Table 8.8. *Excerpt from a computer-aided psychiatric treatment plan using the functional level approach*

INTERVENTIONS
Aggravating Stresses
Problem (P)
P–A1. Minor violation of law
　Short-Term Goal (STG) 1: Obtain necessary legal assistance
　　Method of Treatment (MT) and Time of Attainment (TA): Social Therapy;
　　Legal counsel, if needed; 5 days; stat
　　　Responsible Person (RP) and Frequency of Contact (FC): Social Worker
　　　(SW); once. Attorney; as needed
　Long-Term Goal (LTG) 1: Clarify nature and extent of problem behavior.
　　Method of Treatment (MT) and Time of Attainment (TA): Individual ther-
　　apy (IT); Cognitive Therapy (CT); Behavior Therapy (BT); until discharge.
　　　Responsible Person (RP) and Frequency of Contact (FC): Primary Thera-
　　　pist (PT); t.i.w.
　LTG 2: Train patient to manage problem behavior.
　　Method of Treatment (MT) and Time of Attainment (TA): Individual ther-
　　apy (IT); Cognitive Therapy (CT); Behavior Therapy; Behavioral milieu
　　therapy, token economy, if available; until discharge
　　　Responsible Person (RP) and Frequency of Contact (FC): Primary thera-
　　　pist (PT); t.i.w.
　LTG 3: Train patient to manage stress.
　　Method of Treatment (MT) and Time of Attainment (TA): Stress Manage-
　　ment Class; until discharge.
　　　Responsible Person (RP) and Frequency of Contact (FC): Occupational
　　　Therapist (OT); t.i.w.
　LTG 4: Provide insight into problem and help patient to apply stress and
　problem behavior management training to own personal situation and
　conduct.
　　Method of Treatment (MT) and Time of Attainment (TA): IT; until
　　discharge.
　　　Responsible Person (RP) and Frequency of Contact (FC): Primary Thera-
　　　pist (PT); t.i.w.
　Other Goals:

Coping Skills
P–C23: Cannot or does not manage medications properly
　STG 1: Assess nature and extent of problem.
　　Method of Treatment (MT) and Time of Attainment (TA): Behavioral test-
　　ing; three days.
　　　Responsible Person (RP) and Frequency of Contact (FC): Nurses; two
　　　sessions.
　LTG 1: Learn simple classification, therapeutic effects, side-effects, interac-
　tions, and precautions of basic psychotropic drugs.
　　Method of Treatment (MT) and Time of Attainment (TA): Medication
　　training; until discharge.
　　　Responsible Person (RP) and Frequency of Contact (FC): Nurse and
　　　pharmacist; Medication Classes, if available; t.i.w.

Table 8.8. *Continued*

INTERVENTIONS
Coping Skills (*cont.*)
LTG 2: Provide insight into problem and help patient to apply medication skill training to own personal situation.
Method of Treatment (MT) and Time of Attainment (TA): IT; until discharge.
Responsible Person (RP) and Frequency of Contact (FC): PT; t.i.w.
Other Goals:

Table 8.9. *Patient care monitoring array using elements from the functional level equation (part of a larger array)*

Patient	Period of treatment	Score					Denominator $(A + B)$ total	Numerator $(C + D + E)$ total
		A	*B*	*C*	*D*	*E*		
Margaret[a]	Entering	1	4	1	4	1	5	6
	One year	1	4	3.5	5.3	4.2	5[a]	13
Robbie[a]	Entering	5.6	5	1	2	2	10.6	5
	One year	1	2.5	1.75	2	2.5	3.5	6.25[a]
Joan	Entering	1	4	1	5.5	1	5	7.5
	One year	1	2	2	6	3	3	11
Brenda	Entering	4	4	1.75	3.5	1	8	6.25
	One year	3.3	2	4.5	5	4.3	5.3	13.8
Lawrence	Entering	5	6	2	4	1	11	7
	One year	1	4	4	5	1.5	5	10.5

[a]Patients with the least-improved numerator $(C + D + E)$ totals and denominator $(A + B)$ totals. These cases are selected for utilization reviews and/or patient care monitoring conferences.

FL-equation data are compiled as part of a large array, as shown in Tables 8.9 and 8.10. Table 8.9 presents data from 5 of the 10 patient case histories used in performing the *FL* equation's reliability and validity studies mentioned earlier in this chapter. Table 8.10 provides computed functional level scores on all 10 patients at the two different periods of their treatment. A *t* test showed that treatment resulted in a significant improvement in the patients' functional levels. Table 4.A.9b presents the microcomputer *t*-test analysis of these data.

Table 8.10. *Patient care and program evaluation data for 10 patients receiving long-term treatment (converted functional level scores computed from the* FL *equation)*

	Converted *FL* (entering treatment)	Converted *FL* (after one year)	Difference
Brenda	6.0	4.4	1.6
Valerie	5.3	2.4	2.9
Alfred	5.5	3.4	2.1
Robbie	6.4	5.0	1.4
Joan	5.2	3.8	1.4
Lawrence	6.2	4.8	1.4
Maria	6.0	3.0	3.0
Margaret[a]	5.4	4.3	1.1[a]
Kevin	5.3	2.8	2.5
Sue	6.2	3.0	3.2

Note: A *t* test was used to evaluate the improvement in the group's performance. It showed that the group as a whole improved significantly ($p < .01$) in treatment.
[a]Patient with the least-improved score selected for study of her case.

Patients' progress in treatment is measured by their changes in scores of all six *A* through *FL* scales, as shown in Marna's case example and in Tables 8.9 and 8.10. Therapists and program directors use these data to monitor the progress of individual patients in every component of their therapy. As discussed in the legends of the two tables, program evaluators can tell at a glance which patients are not progressing satisfactorily, and in which of their five predictor areas they still have problems. They can then implement necessary changes.

Reviewing professional performance

Individual professionals, clinical programs, and mental health departments often receive responsibility for specific elements in patient care. Individual therapists treat a number of patients; rehabilitation personnel usually help patients improve their coping skills; and social workers manage environmental supports. In facilities where these roles are clarified, the individual therapist's or whole department's performance with a group of patients can be appraised quantitatively with the help of a microcomputer.

The examples using pooled data from a number of patients show that the *FL* equation can be used to plan psychiatric treatment and to upgrade programs by controlling the variables that affect them. Software programs for the personal computer simplify analyses of individual patients' and pooled groups' scores. They promote evaluation of treatment programs, monitoring of patient care, review of resource utilization and performance of staff, and other quality assurance procedures.

DSM-III-R *and psychiatric insurance*

Clinical psychiatrists and the American Psychiatric Association have been concerned about cutbacks and inequities in psychiatric insurance coverage. They have been focusing their efforts on obtaining nondiscriminatory coverage for psychiatric illness in the legislative and public affairs arenas. However, the APA's revised diagnostic manual *DSM-III-R* may provide them with a new, scientific approach to this goal. Based on our research experience with *DSM-III*'s multiaxial system discussed in this book, we propose that *DSM-III-R* may provide data for quantitative analysis of patients' treatment needs and benefits that can be used in a rational approach to insuring and monitoring psychiatric care.

We have shown how *DSM-III*'s multiaxial system can be useful in five areas – planning hospitalization of psychiatric patients, predicting their treatment needs, measuring their response to treatment, evaluating the outcome of treatment programs, and comparing patients and facilities in different areas of the country. Studies like these with *DSM-III-R*'s new, expanded quantitative measures may provide data to enable psychiatric insurers to develop nondiscriminatory insurance based on sound actuarial evidence.

DSM-III-R *'s modified multiaxial system*

The revised *DSM-III-R* expanded multiaxial system may simplify the quantitative analysis of patients' needs and their responses to psychiatric treatment. It contains modifications of Axes IV and V and a new specification of *current severity of disorder*. The Axes IV and V modifications include (1) a division of the aggravating stressors in Axis IV into predominantly acute events (precipitators of less than six months' duration) and predominantly enduring circumstances (pressurizers of greater than six months' duration) and (2) a new Axis V scale for global assessment of functioning that will be used to measure not only premorbid functioning but also current functioning.

The researches described above have pointed to the importance of assessing severity and of measuring current as well as premorbid functional level. You might also consider assessing both acute stressors (precipitators) and enduring ones (pressurizers) on Axis IV with the new *DSM-III* system. The former can be expected to respond more quickly to therapy than the latter.

Psychiatrists and psychiatric facilities will need to test our observations in their own settings (where nonclinical variables, such as amount of insurance coverage available, do not interfere with patients' *LOS*). If the tests confirm the findings, insurers will have data with which to determine whether patients' length of inpatient care is appropriate. They also will be able to estimate which patients will need lengthy care and which can be handled in brief periods of hospitalization. In writing individual psychiatric insurance policies they may be able to charge premiums that reflect the psychiatric risks involved in the same manner as they do with policies for physical disorders.

New causal relation research

Previous sections have treated functional level (*FL*) both as a correlated observed relation variable (for example, in predicting length of hospital stay) and as a dependent observed causal variable (for example, in measuring outcome of treatment). We have provided research data that showed how it can serve both these purposes.

However, when used to improve treatment planning, performance of professional staff, and the quality of care of groups of patients, *FL* can become an independent variable in causal relation research. Our hypothesis is that the *FL* approach to treatment planning leads to more cost-effective and efficient care of patients. Patients understand better what treatment is accomplishing as they participate in developing their *FL*-based treatment plans. Professional staff provide more comprehensive and more efficient care of patients when they systematically attend to all six components of the equation. Patients and professionals then work more actively to improve patients' *FL*s (the independent variable) by increasing their coping skills, directive power, and environmental supports and reducing their aggravating stresses and biomedical impairments (the mediating variables). An experimental group of patients using the *FL* treatment plan approach should respond better and more efficiently than a matched control group who use a traditional treatment plan, as measured by the experimental group's requiring less time in treatment, less expense, and less hospital care (the dependent variables) to raise its mean functional level to a predetermined level.

This hypothesis can be tested in experimental causal relation studies. We are now preparing to conduct such research, and we welcome efforts of others to do so too.

Publishing

Rather than waiting for acceptance from refereed journals, we published early papers on the functional level theory in a district branch newsletter (Alderman et al., 1984; R. E. Gordon & Gordon, 1982). This gave priority of publication over others who may have been thinking about and working with a similar formulation related to Albee's thesis. Further, we also kept our copyright, rather than surrendering it to an outside journal. Meanwhile, we submitted reports of other data to major specialty journals and as a chapter of a book. These were published more than a year after the copyrighted versions first appeared.

Summary

This chapter has advanced a theory that brings together the main quantifiable variables in psychiatric practice and treatment into one formula: $FL = f(C + D + E)/(A + B)$. The components of this FL equation can be assessed by means of rating scales. The theory has stimulated a number of research studies. Findings from these show that the FL equation can be used to (1) classify rating scales, goals in treatment, staff roles, types of facilities, and variables in research studies; (2) predict length of hospital treatment needed and differences between symptomatic response and functional response to therapy; and (3) control efforts to enhance a patient's functional level in treatment planning and to improve the quality of treatment programs.

9. Research ethics

This addresses some of the ethical matters you must consider when conducting psychiatric and other medical researches. It discusses eight categories of problems: (1) conducting poorly controlled research; (2) bending the data; (3) providing new therapies; (4) performing potentially harmful or painful studies; (5) getting cooperation from colleagues; (6) citing others; (7) giving credit to collaborators; and (8) obtaining financial support from concerns with vested interests.

Conducting poorly controlled research

It is often impossible to conduct clinical research that is as rigorous as you would like. Costs, time pressures, and other practical considerations often lead to cutting corners, reducing the number of subjects, using poorly selected controls, or taking other shortcuts that fit the realities of the situation. When such work gets published, it may remain in the literature of the field for a long time until someone comes along and repeats the study under better-controlled conditions. When the new results contradict earlier findings, not only does someone's research reputation suffer, but many patients and therapists have wasted their time, energy, and funds following a path that led nowhere.

It is a far better and safer policy to refer to the initial observed causal research as a preliminary study, and to redo the investigation as soon as possible, using appropriate rigor. Bear in mind that once a research is printed it is part of the permanent literature. Colleagues make use of the findings only to discover that their patients do not react the way yours seem to.

In accordance with this rule, the less rigorous quasi-experimental combined treatment studies were followed up with new, more rigorous investigations into the various components of the preliminary work. The sub-

214

sequent researches on preventing postpartum distress, modular psychoeducation, and reducing rehospitalization all reevaluated the innovative aspects of the earlier studies – managing behavior, training coping skills, providing peer and other supports – under better-controlled conditions.

Bending data

Sometimes, after months of hard work, the results turn out to be inconclusive, or perhaps contrary to the hypothesis. This may bring on an urge to bend the data a little so that there will be significant results to report. But the data do not really bend. At some time in the future, the error will turn up. Sometimes a disappointed researcher will simply apply a different statistic that does show the difference expected in the first place. But if the new statistic is inappropriate, using it accomplishes nothing.

Keep in mind that your reputation is on the line when you report research results. You are breaking new ground and contributing to the scientific lore in your field. You owe it to yourself, your colleagues, the scientific community at large, and the patients who will – or will not – benefit from your work to adhere as closely as possible to the tenets of objective, scientific executing and reporting of the study.

Therefore, the more qualified subjects you can include, the more exactly you can define your variables, and the more care you can exercise in analyzing the results, the better. And if, after all that, your study turns out to have no significant results, then the course of wisdom is to accept the fact and go at the problem from a different viewpoint.

Providing new therapies or tests

When patients enter new treatment or testing programs where there may be potential risks or discomforts, there is an elaborate procedure for obtaining permission from the hospital's human subjects research review board, and for asking for informed consent from the patients involved. Further, when new, improved treatment methods are introduced, as in our studies on preventing postpartum distress, reducing rehospitalization, and modular psychoeducation, it is often a disadvantage to be a control subject who receives only traditional care. Therefore it is necessary to obtain patients' permission to serve voluntarily in this kind of study. The same consideration also applies when there is reason to doubt that the new therapy will be effective.

Obtaining permission from patients

Whenever you perform a controlled research into new methods of testing or treatment, you must obtain permission from the patients in the study. They must fill in informed-consent forms and agree in writing to participate.

An informed-consent form must contain the following elements: (1) a description of the benefits to be expected; (2) a description of the potential discomforts or risks; (3) a description of alternative services that might prove equally advantageous to them; (4) a full explanation of the procedures to be followed, especially those that are experimental in nature; (5) a statement that the participants' right to privacy and confidentiality will be protected; (6) a clause stating that a patient's refusal to participate in a research project will not be a cause for denying services the patient may need; (7) a sentence that allows participants to withdraw consent and discontinue participation in the research project at any time without affecting their status in the program; and (8) a statement that the investigators will adhere to the ethical standards of their professions, and that they will be guided by the regulations of the U.S. Department of Health and Human Services and all other federal, state, and local statutes and regulations concerning the protection of human subjects.

On the other hand, studies may provide you with new, nonaversive therapies such as psychoeducational treatment, behavior management, social supports, and so on. You may begin to treat all new patients with them as soon as possible, and use as comparison groups those patients who were treated previously by acceptable standard methods that were then available. The combined treatment study (see chapter 6) was in this category. The research consisted essentially of reviewing patients' records and evaluating how effective the new treatment approaches were as compared with the previous ones. Although the research showed that the comparison groups, who had been treated previously, had been at a disadvantage, there was little that could be done about it other than to provide the comparison patients with the new, improved treatment approach if they returned for further therapy.

When you conduct a retrospective program evaluation by review of your own or a hospital's charts, as in the combined treatment study, you do not need to obtain informed consent from the patients. You are subjecting them to no unusual new treatments and are causing them no possible pain or harm. You must only keep all identifiers – patients' names, social security numbers, and other personal information – confidential.

The combined treatment patients did not fill in permission forms unless their specific case histories were described in a report.

The effectiveness of the new treatment approaches was reported in the medical literature, in articles in popular magazines and books, and in presentations at medical meetings. If old patients who had not received the new techniques and had served in the comparison groups were referred or returned for further therapy, they were treated with the new methods of care.

These same principles apply to researches into the usefulness of new tests. If you perform a controlled prospective measurement research study, you will need to obtain informed consent from both the experimental and control patients/subjects. On the other hand, retrospective chart reviews of the benefits of new tests as compared with old ones do not require patients' consent. The retrospective measurement research studies of psychiatric inpatients and outpatients on whom complete multiaxial *Diagnostic and Statistical Manual for Mental Disorders* (*DSM-III*) diagnoses had been made were in this category. These studies of the usefulness and validity of Axes IV and V were exempted by the hospital's human research review board from the need to obtain informed consent as long as patient identifiers were kept confidential.

Obtaining approval from authorities

Obtaining permission for studies conducted in college and other institutional settings may differ to some extent from getting permission for those performed in your office. The students who were the subjects of our researches either were required to undergo periodic complete physical and laboratory examinations (football players and student nurses) or were enrolled in psychology courses in which they were required to participate as subjects in a research project.

To perform research with their academic and biochemical data required that approval be obtained for the study from the college administration and that personal information be kept confidential. To obtain records of college students' laboratory test findings and academic progress, you cannot merely ask for them in the same way you can visit the patient record room of the hospital where you are privileged to serve on the staff. You must obtain permission from those in authority. This will require that you present a written description of your proposed research for their study and approval.

Performing painful or potentially harmful studies

Ethical considerations interfere with your experimenting with most path-ogenic influences, such as imposing overwhelming stresses on humans, creating brain lesions, or administering toxic chemicals, without the informed consent of volunteers. Who can obtain such volunteers in a pri-vate psychiatric practice, or elsewhere? How would you go about getting women to participate in a causal relation research on the benefits of resisting rape? The researches reported in the literature on the long-term effects upon human health of habitually smoking tobacco are all observed relation studies. To perform a controlled experiment where nonsmoking humans are randomly assigned to smoke-exposed and smoke-free groups would not be tolerated in a free society. Usually all that can be done with humans is to examine the correlations between various diseases and numbers of cigarettes smoked daily over time by habitual smokers and persons, such as family, who are exposed to them.

You can sometimes measure findings in naturalistic observations such as by studying relationships between the stress of the football season and players' serum chemicals, or by comparing the numbers of diseases and the life expectancy of persons who live with smokers – such as their spouses and children, and especially the infants born to smoking moth-ers – with figures for persons who do not. You can usually perform prop-erly controlled studies to test pathogens by experimenting with animals, usually white mice or rats. But recently animal liberation groups have objected to the use of primates for brain-behavior observed relation stud-ies. Sometimes they succeed in placing a referendum on the ballot to for-bid vivisection of all vertebrates. Human rights advocates in Florida have prevented the postmortem study, without prior informed consent, of tissues from the brains of executed murderers for evidence of possible links between previous brain lesions and criminal violence, even though the law requires autopsies of all executed criminals.

Getting cooperation from patients and colleagues

Try to plan your data collection to be as efficient and as unobtrusive to patients as possible and to maintain the good will of professional col-leagues and ward, laboratory, and record room staff. Schedule your data collection in advance and at times when you will not interfere with staff in the performance of their routine duties. Either collect the data yourself or arrange for someone in your employ or collaborating with you to do so. Do not expect others to put aside their primary duties in order to collect your data if you want to obtain trustworthy results and avoid bothering busy staff and creating ill will toward yourself and your research.

The maternity questionnaire study and the study on preventing post-partum distress needed the cooperation of 45 obstetricians in private practice to rate their maternity patients' emotional condition. These and other studies also worked with nurses, hospital and clinic record room personnel, and others, none of whom received compensation for their efforts. In general, it was fairly easy to obtain professional colleagues' and others' assistance when they understood in advance the nature of the research, why it might be important to them and their patients, and that they would need to perform only small chores. Ninety-six percent of the obstetricians in the psychiatric maternity studies scored over 3,000 brief ratings on over 500 women at three different time periods.

Always be sure to report back on what you found to the professionals and staff who worked with you, and be sure to give them credit in your publications. They appreciate the courtesy, and readily welcome you back the next time you want to study their patients. They may also volunteer to join you as coresearchers in subsequent studies. Also report back to patients and other subjects on the findings of the studies in which they participated. The football players and other college students upon whom the serum chemical studies were performed were quite interested in their cholesterol and uric acid test results, since high serum chemical levels are potential warning signs of later heart and other diseases.

Citing others' studies

Be sure to give credit to authors whose work led to or was related to yours. Look at the citations in the journal where you plan to submit, and use the same format in your references. There are no hard-and-fast rules about length of quotations; in general, you may quote short passages without obtaining permission in a review, critique, or scholarly or technical article to illustrate, clarify, or comment on a point. For lengthier excerpts, contact the author and copyright holder for permission.

If you have any questions, consult your librarian. To avoid ill feeling and possible accusations of plagiarism, it is wise to err on the side of citing others and of getting permission to quote them. Even when you show a table or other illustration from one of your own publications, you must nowadays ask the publishers for permission if they hold the copyright. In our experience, they invariably give it, but you still need to ask. (This is one of the reasons we sometimes submit articles to publications like our district branch newsletter where we can keep our copyright.)

Giving credit where credit is due

This topic is important enough to receive its own section. Many people often enter into the creative process that results in a good piece of research. For those who are strictly employees and who are paid for the time they spend doing routine tasks connected with the study, there is no need for further remuneration beyond their salaries and a few words of recognition at the end of your report. But for those who contribute ideas, research designs, methods of analysis, and insights into the meaning of the results, some recompense in keeping with the importance of these contributions is appropriate – and necessary if you expect to work with them again.

For example, if you make use of members of the faculty of a college or university for substantive consultation or other help in conducting the research, coauthorship of the completed study is appropriate compensation. Academic currency is counted in number and quality of publications. When faculty members are working on your research, they are not spending time on their own, which may be to their detriment if they cannot share in the glory of publishing your work. Of course names should never be added to a publication without the permission of the persons involved. They may have reasons for not wanting their names on your report. These details should be worked out ahead of time when you first seek consultation with the faculty members.

Here again you will build your reputation in the scientific community according to the courtesy and respect you accord to those who work for and with you on such projects. If you expect to do more research in the future, it will be to your advantage to share the benefits of it with those who made a substantial contribution to the work.

In some settings, the name of the head of the organization or department is routinely entered as one of the coauthors, whether or not that person even knew the research was being conducted. This is an unfortunate practice; it diminishes the importance of honest contributions to the research. It unnecessarily glorifies someone whose real abilities may be in administration, fund raising, handling the day-to-day paper work of an organization, or political machinations, rather than in creating research-able ideas or in determining how to investigate a patient problem in a manner that will be generalizable to other patients. Wherever possible, this approach to sharing the benefits of research should be avoided. There are other rewards available to competent administrators. Research is a field in itself, and those who are adept at it should receive acknowledg-ment of their contribution in terms of an appropriately ranked listing among the coauthors.

Obtaining financial support from vested interests

Occasionally the manufacturer of a product may be willing to support a scientific study of the possible benefits of his product. (In the case of drugs, of course, it is mandatory that the product be tested by indepen-dent laboratories.) Manufacturers of products where outside testing is not mandatory often feel that a product will benefit from an endorsement by a member of the medical profession. In this case, what the manufacturer really wants is to have you perform some test that will show the product's benefits.

From your standpoint, however, the test must be one that will deter-mine from an objective viewpoint whether or not the product has any benefit. This is sometimes a hard line to hold. Here is where the design of the experiment is of utmost importance. There is a vast difference between a demonstration of the product's benefits and an experimental test of its efficacy. Resisting the manufacturer's blandishments will be easier if you have a firm grasp of the principles of research and can state with confidence that a specified number of control groups are required, along with a predetermined number of subjects who must be tested on a certain number of trials over a minimum amount of time.

Any other type of test – that is, the demonstration that the manufac-turer wants – may threaten your reputation. Worse still, if the products can actually have dangerous effects, you may both harm the patients who use them and place your professional career in jeopardy. If you conduct research for a manufacturer, be sure to transmit your report to him in writing so that there can be no question about what results you obtained and whether or not you are endorsing the product.

These are some of the considerations to keep in mind when you are approached by someone who might profit financially from the results of your research. In specific situations, there may be many other pitfalls. Therefore legal advice and a tightly written contract for the work may be advisable.

Summary

Chapter 9 has discussed eight kinds of potential ethical problems that arise in performing research.

10. Summary and conclusions

What to look for in journal articles

Determining the type of research

When reading a research report in a journal, keep in mind the stage or rank of the study. Is it research to formulate an initial working hypothesis? Research to develop measuring instruments? Observed relation research? Observed causal research? Causal relation research? Or theory development?

An *initial hypothesis* is just an idea, no matter how much it appeals to you. Before you can believe that the author has gotten hold of a piece of important truth, you must see supportive data from patients. This means that he or she or someone else must do quantitative research to prove its value before you can risk using it on your patients. This brings us to the first level of quantification – developing measuring instruments.

Measurement research must show that the concept or hypothesis can be measured and that the tests or instruments for measuring it are valid, reliable, sensitive, and selective. Psychiatry would like to use more of the physical, chemical, and physiological – hard science – tests that other medical specialties employ. This accounts for the great enthusiasm over new biochemical assays and graphic physical measures. But most of these still are awaiting evidence that, except for some limited uses, they are reliable, valid, and not too costly. Psychiatric scales and tests present a different problem. Many are standardized, but they are limited in their scope – measuring only psychopathology, for instance, and not patients' needs, strengths, skills, and supports. Psychiatry needs more comprehensive tests or combinations of instruments, like those under investigation in research on the functional level equation, which measure all or most of the major factors in patients' functioning.

In studies at the stage of *observed relation research,* watch out that the author does not claim or infer more than the data allow. Numerous reports imply causality between an observation and a diagnosis when the data only show a correlation. Both may be caused by something else that the researcher did not control. The same is true for *observed causal studies.* They can lead to erroneous conclusions unless followed by well-controlled *causal relation studies.*

Determining the quality of the research

Consider the rigor with which the research was conducted. Note how many subjects were used. Some journals still print research conducted on two or three subjects with no effort to assess the implications of the results. Although studies using only a few subjects have value in calling attention to unusual cases, realize that you cannot extrapolate directly from such work to your own patients. Statistics and groups of subjects are used in creditable research in order to cancel out the effects of individual differences between subjects. When very few subjects are used, the individual differences may be so large that what worked on those subjects will have no effect on your patients.

Look for precise descriptions of the populations used as subjects. If the study states only that 10 women were in each group, without any qualifications about the age range, marital status, symptomatology, or other defining characteristics of the women, then you have no idea what population the study refers to, or whether or not the subjects are comparable with your female patients.

Notice the characteristics of the control group. Does the author state that these were matched controls, or that each subject was used as his or her own control, or that he or she simply used a comparison group? You need to know how well the controls matched the experimental group in order to know if the author's significant difference between groups has any significance for your purposes.

Read carefully what methods the author used to get the results. Is there a chance for experimenter bias in the way the study was conducted? If it is not clear from the author's methods section just how he went about conducting the study, then there is no basis for giving credence to the results.

Examining the statistics

In the past, many psychiatrists have shied away from statistics. Editors sometimes have deleted the statistics from articles submitted to their journals, fearing that mentioning chi-squares and probabilities would scare away psychiatric readers. Now they often request that psychiatric researchers supply further quantitative details.

Determine first how the researcher's data are scaled. Did the author use an appropriate statistical procedure; for example, nonparametrics for nominal and ordinal-scaled data, parametrics only for interval or ratio-scaled data? Remember that you can use nonparametrics with ordinal, interval, and ratio-scaled data (though you will lose power by doing so) but must never use parametrics with nominal or ordinal-scaled data.

Look at the statistical significance the author claims for the results obtained. A probability of the statistic showing the result by chance should be stated in the article, e.g. "$p < .05$" or "$p < .01$." If such a probability is not stated at all, then you have no basis for putting any faith in the study regardless of how convincing the rest of the article may be. Wait for more definitive results to be announced or try to replicate the study yourself before giving credence to it.

With any of the points above, the fault may lie in the writing of the article, in the conduct of the study, or both. Editors do not always catch inadequacies in research reports. Therefore, if the work may have some direct importance to your own research or to the conduct of your own practice, feel free to correspond with the author and ask him these questions. Authors are always interested in knowing that their work has been read and will usually be glad to answer questions about it.

Practicing scientific psychiatry in your office and hospital

Clinicians in most medical specialties routinely use radiograms and physiological, pathological, and biochemical tests to demonstrate objectively the nature of the patient's problem and the effectiveness of their treatments. Chest X rays document the exact location and extent of the medical patient's pneumonitis and its response to therapy. Blood pressure or sugar levels provide measures of patient response to treatment. Pathologists examine specimens removed in surgical operations to determine the initial size of the patient's tumor and whether it has been fully extirpated. No wonder internal medicine, radiology, pathology, and surgery are highly respected and well-paid specialties. They practice much of the science of medicine as well as the art.

Performing initial assessments and collecting objective data in clinical practice

To practice scientific psychiatry in your office and hospital care of patients, use quantitative precision in collecting data and assessing each patient's needs, strengths, problems, and subsequent course in therapy. Obtain objective data about patients' lives and progress like those described in the studies of the effects of new patient treatment approaches described in chapters 6–8 – information about their history of psychiatric care, their success at work and school, their arrests, their marriages and divorces, and so forth. Include standardized clinical interview schedules such as the Diagnostic Interview Schedule (DIS) (Robins, Helzer, Croughan & Ratcliff, 1981). Try to make every bit of information collected from the patient a reliable and valid potential research datum. When insurance companies question your charges, you will have quantitative information to report to them about your patient's needs, what you did about them, and how the patient responded. Use objective diagnoses like those in *DSM-III* and standardized tests as much as possible, tests on which norms have been obtained with thousands of patients. Then you can show in the manner described in chapter 8 how much your patients have improved in their test results as compared with others with the same problems.

The revised *DSM-III-R* (American Psychiatric Association, 1987) multiaxial system may turn out to be very helpful to you in this process. If studies on the usefulness of its quantitative scales confirm the *DSM-III* findings, it may be worth your while to use all five axes in diagnosing new patients. This may provide you with data that would allow you early in their treatment to determine quantitatively (1) their diagnosis and treatment needs, (2) their need for special care like hospitalization, (3) the approximate length of stay they would require, (4) the amount of time and approximate number of outpatient treatment sessions they would need. Furthermore, if you assess current functional level with the Axis V scale, as well as premorbid functional level, you may be able use the former as an objective outcome measure. If you decide later to conduct a retrospective program evaluation and to determine the outcome of your treatment with a group of patients in the manner described in this book, you would have easily retrievable quantitative data with which to work.

The personal computer greatly simplifies this process. We showed examples of microcomputer statistical analyses for assessing patients with tests and scales in chapters 4.A and 5.A and elsewhere in this book. The functional level equation, which complements *DSM-III,* is being prepared for use with the personal computer.

In addition to using standardized psychiatric rating scales with your patients, obtain neuropsychological assessments when appropriate, and biochemical analyses and physical tests such as nuclear magnetic resonance images, topographic brain maps, and computer-aided tomographs. Research is pointing to brain areas and neurotransmitters that are related to rage, pleasure, panic, and possibly obsessions and compulsions. Disorders in some of these may respond to psychopharmaceuticals and other treatments. Before relying upon a new test to measure anatomical, biochemical, or physiological abnormalities, find out first about its reliability and validity, since many promising new procedures have turned out to be unreliable, to have low validity, and to be inordinately costly.

Bear in mind that physical and biochemical tools can only assess biomedical impairments. The aggravating stresses burdening patients, the coping skills they utilize, the directive power they exercise over people and material resources, and the environmental supports available to them are at present measured best with objective psychiatric rating scales and tests. Although body responses to stress can be assessed physiologically, the reliability and validity of these measures are often questionable. Many researchers are looking for chemical, electroencephalographic, and other physiological correlates of aspects of psychiatric disease and behavior, but no one is likely to find a way to measure social skills with a brain scan or environmental supports with a biochemical test.

In other words, the pathological, radiological, biochemical, and physiological laboratories provide measuring instruments for practicing scientific medicine and surgery, but they can contribute only to a small extent to the practice of scientific psychiatry. Objective psychosocial tests and instruments are the most useful tools for the clinical psychiatrist. These tests require only a modest understanding and use of the simple statistics discussed in this book to assess patients and measure their response to treatment.

Planning treatment and measuring progress in therapy

Handle every treatment like a research project. Try to systematize your treatment plans in a manner like that used in the functional level approach, so that the data are comparable and statistically analyzable. Follow up on your treatment plans by measuring patients' progress in therapy on appropriate, reliable, and valid psychiatric tests and scales. Use statistical procedures to determine whether the patients are improving significantly.

Assuring quality

Perform your own quality assurance. Examine each patient's test results to find out which problems have not yet responded to therapy. Change your treatment accordingly. Keep permanent quantitative records on all your patients. Periodically pool and review the data. Determine whether there are trends in the kinds of patients who are consulting you, or in their needs, or in their responses to your care.

Conducting follow-ups

You may wish to invite your patients to continue to see you every six months even after they have recovered from the acute phase of their illnesses (R. E. Gordon, 1966). Besides the therapeutic benefits to the patients, there is another benefit from seeing your patients periodically: You can follow up on the continued effectiveness of your care by quantitatively assessing their progress years after they initiated treatment with you.

Even if you do not see them after you have discharged them from treatment, you can keep in touch by mail, sending them birthday and holiday cards and periodically including brief questionnaires to obtain follow-up information on their psychiatric status. When you have thousands of former patients to whom to write each year, the costs in time and money will be compensated for by the return visits of those who need further treatment. And you will have an invaluable supply of subjects for follow-up clinical research.

The microcomputer can also help you here. Each day it can provide you with the names and addresses of patients whose birthdays are current. It will even print out gummed labels for your envelopes.

Performing peer review

If you are called upon to conduct peer reviews, you can apply the same quantitative perspective to the review of your colleagues' work. Do they use quantitative assessments that contribute to the patients' diagnostic assessments? Are their assessments comprehensive in measuring every important component of the patients' needs and problems? Can their treatments be assessed statistically to show whether they are effective? Can they demonstrate objectively the requirement for certain procedures? Are they using cost-effective and efficient standardized testing and treatment procedures or unreliable, expensive ones of questionable validity? Do they present evidence of why the patients are or are not improving?

Evaluating new tests and treatments

When you try out a new test or therapy, try to design a study with controls, or at least with some kind of comparison group. Try to obtain community norms for your tests, or conduct studies of normals, as was done with normal maternity patients. Compare the findings under the new procedure statistically with those under the previous one, and determine whether the new is significantly better than the old.

Assessing the patients in your practice

Compare your patients' needs and characteristics with those obtained from community epidemiological surveys. Do the data agree? Have you discovered a special new group of patients like the orbiting veterans? Should you change your treatment program to meet the new group's needs?

Improving patient care

Keep upgrading your treatments to match the needs of your patients. And keep monitoring your results. This is easy with a personal computer. Continually feed back the findings from your studies into the care of your patients.

Serving on a quality assurance committee

If you are appointed to one of a clinic's or hospital's quality assurance committees – for doing needs assessment, patient care monitoring, peer review, program evaluation, or utilization review, for example – insist upon a high standard of scientific rigor in the way your group conducts its studies.

Assessing the needs of patients in the program

Determine the general needs of the specific patients the program is treating, needs that differ for children, younger adults, and the elderly, for specialty and for general hospitals, and so on. Obtain data from epidemiological observed relation surveys of your community, or perform your own patient needs assessments, to find out what your specific patient group may need. Are there large numbers of elderly newcomers with truncated social supports? Are alcoholism and substance abuse major problems among the youth? Periodically perform new assessments of the characteristics of the patients who come to your program.

Monitoring patient care

Use your quantitative assessments to determine whether individual patients are progressing satisfactorily in treatment. If not, try to find out what happened or failed to happen to those who did not progress satisfactorily, as we try to do with the five scales of the functional level equation.

Reviewing utilization

If you find yourself in a position to influence the review process, try to make it become more systematic and precise. Procedures for assessing whether patients needed admission to the hospital, whether they are remaining for too long or too short a period in treatment, whether they received too many or too few tests or medications, and so forth can be made more scientific. When the nature and severity of patients' conditions are documented with standardized tests and their data are compared with those of other patients and norms, it will be clearer whether their care consumed greater or fewer resources than necessary.

Evaluating programs

Are your hospital's programs effective? Can you prove it? Researches such as the evaluations of veterans', chronic mental, and private psychiatric patients' programs discussed in this book enable you to collect data that will help you to answer these questions. Perform these and show them to the team from the Joint Commission on Accreditation of Hospitals when next they survey your program. They will be favorably impressed.

Directing hospital or clinic programs

If you are in a position of control as director of a program in a hospital or clinic, you are in a position to implement rigorously scientific procedures throughout your unit or section. And you can apply the same approaches to personal practice. Further, if you get an idea about a new treatment, you can consider performing a research to test it.

Conducting research studies

There is nothing complicated about reporting a new hypothesis. You need no help from a consultant to review the literature thoroughly, put down your ideas, and send them to a journal that prints related articles.

If you decide to test your hypothesis in a measurement, observed relation, or causal relation study, it is usually a good idea first to follow up your literature review with a retrospective study, if possible, of your own or your hospital's patient records. You can also do this without any extra help from an expert. You have no control over the variables in a retrospective study, since the events occurred before you did the research, but you can still determine with minimal effort whether the new measurement instrument discriminated significantly between patients with the condition and those free from it; or whether there was a significant relationship among the patients in your files between certain historical and behavioral characteristics; or whether your new medication or other treatment improved the symptoms of a certain diagnostic group of patients significantly more than did the treatment previously used.

Retrospective studies do not take much time or expense; they provide preliminary evidence as to whether your hypothesis is worth pursuing further. If there are no significant differences between the groups in your retrospective study, there may be no point in going further. If there are differences, then you can feel justified in putting in the greater effort required to perform a prospective research. Write up and report your findings and begin designing a prospective study where you can control the important variables.

Using a consultant

You will need to write up your research proposal for the facility management's approval. Here you might begin to consider calling for some assistance from a consultant in research design or statistics. If you are planning to submit a request for funding, it is always a good idea to go over your plan with a consultant. Questions of numbers of subjects – experimentals and controls, matching, and so on – are best answered with the help of a professional with considerable experience in clinical research design.

If you are considering using any statistics, let a statistician decide what to use. Let the professional handle this part of the research for you, at least until you have gained considerable experience with the statistics chosen. Even if you have a computer and the statistical software to analyze the data, let a statistician decide which statistical program is most appropriate and what is the best method of compiling the data.

Consult with an expert if you decide not to use a standardized questionnaire or test but need to develop your own instrument. Then you will learn how to handle details of establishing reliability and validity of the instrument.

You will need patient permission forms. And you will need to determine whether you can conduct a full-scale controlled experiment or whether you must content yourself with a quasi-experimental observed causal preliminary project. The latter approach is not a bad idea; if you get promising results in the preliminary study, you can generally get support for following up with a well-controlled one.

If you take the step from an observed causal research to a full-scale controlled causal relation experiment, you may need two units – one for the patients whom you have randomly selected to be experimentals and one for those whom you have selected to be controls. (Bear in mind that the patients must not be self-selected unless you control for this.) You will also need to train staff in the new experimental procedures. (But they will have been learning in the quasi-experimental phase of the study.) You may also want to transfer staff at the midpoint of the experiment and reassign those working with control patients to work with experimentals and vice versa. Then differences among staff members will not be so likely to account for the statistical differences you obtain in your research findings.

Practicing scientific psychiatry in court appearances

As your patient's physician

As your patient's psychiatrist, your testimony consists of your professional scientific evaluation of your patient. Your diagnosis of your patient's condition, your treatment, and your prognosis may be contradicted by a psychiatrist hired by the other side wielding an impressive battery of psychosocial, physical, biochemical, and physiological tests performed on your patient. Therefore, it is well for you also to gather and present as much scientific factual information, like that discussed in this book, as possible.

As an expert witness

In this capacity, you do not necessarily represent the side of the court case (plaintiff or defendant) who hired you; you represent your field of expertise. Your function is to edify the court and the jury in the details of a specialty with which the lay public may not be familiar. For example, if you appear as an expert witness in rape trials, arm yourself with data and statistics like those shown in Tables 5.6 and 5.7. Present the facts of what happens to women who try to fight their assailants and other pertinent data. If called upon by hospital groups to determine community needs for psychiatric beds, gather and present data like those shown in Tables 5.3 and 5.4.

In court situations there is an almost overwhelming tendency to be a human being first and an expert witness second. Just as you rarely watch a football game without cheering for one side, you may be tempted to enter a courtroom hoping that your side will win. However, it is necessary for the sake of one's own reputation, and for that of one's field of scientific expertise, to embrace objectivity and eschew partiality to the highest degree possible. Presenting research data will enable you to do this.

Influencing public policy

If you have a good idea about how to improve patients' care nationally, you can avoid tragic effects upon patients by first conducting a well-controlled study demonstrating the value of your proposed program. Psychiatrists played a major role in the national policy decision that shifted many chronically ill mental patients from the wards of the nation's state hospitals onto the streets of its cities. Little preliminary research had shown whether America's deinstitutionalized chronic mentally ill could manage, or even survive, outside mental hospitals (Wyatt, 1986). Research that determined what skills and social supports they needed was done after the national crisis had resulted. The presence today of thousands of the homeless mentally ill on our nation's city streets not only is a tragedy for the patients themselves but also does much harm to the public image of psychiatry.

Psychiatrists today are speaking out before governmental bodies on other important issues where there is little psychiatric or other scientific research evidence to support a position – on adoptions and on immigration policies, among others. You may be in a position to affect important public decisions in your state or nationally. If so, we suggest that you ask policy makers first to obtain research data before making a major change like emptying out the psychiatric hospitals. Or do the studies yourself. This book has shown how to conduct the needs assessments and evaluation researches required.

Conclusion

There is no doubt that the variables with which the psychiatrist must work are not easy to measure or predict. Yet if psychiatrists are to achieve and maintain a credible position in the hierarchy of modern medical practitioners, they must measure and predict. Fortunately at this time the methods and the logic are in place for psychiatry to follow the same route that other branches of medicine have done. What is lacking more than anything else is the realization by the practitioners of the specialty that it will take this kind of rigor to establish clinical psychiatry as a science.

Scientific method, embodied in the principles espoused in this book, has come late to psychiatry, as it has to most of the social sciences. But it offers hope for understanding and controlling the variables with which psychiatrists – and their patients – must cope every day. This book has shown you the methods and tools of psychiatric science and provided you with examples of how to use them.

Appendix

Table A.1. Table of critical values of chi-square

df							Probability							
	.995	.990	.975	.95	.90	.75	.50	.25	.10	.05	.025	.010	.005	.001
1	$.0^4393$	$.0^3157$	$.0^3982$	$.0^2393$	.0158	0.102	0.455	1.323	2.706	3.841	5.024	6.635	7.879	10.83
2	.0100	.0201	.0506	0.103	0.211	0.575	1.386	2.773	4.605	5.991	7.378	9.210	10.60	13.82
3	.0717	0.115	0.216	0.352	0.584	1.213	2.366	4.108	6.251	7.815	9.348	11.34	12.84	16.27
4	0.207	0.297	0.484	0.711	1.064	1.923	3.357	5.385	7.779	9.488	11.14	13.28	14.86	18.47
5	0.412	0.554	0.831	1.145	1.610	2.675	4.351	6.626	9.236	11.07	12.83	15.09	16.75	20.52
6	0.676	0.872	1.237	1.635	2.204	3.455	5.348	7.841	10.64	12.59	14.45	16.81	18.55	22.46
7	0.989	1.239	1.690	2.167	2.833	4.255	6.346	9.037	12.02	14.07	16.01	18.48	20.28	24.32
8	1.344	1.646	2.180	2.733	3.490	5.071	7.344	10.22	13.36	15.51	17.53	20.09	21.95	26.12
9	1.735	2.088	2.700	3.325	4.168	5.899	8.343	11.39	14.68	16.92	19.02	21.67	23.59	27.88
10	2.156	2.558	3.247	3.940	4.865	6.737	9.342	12.55	15.99	18.31	20.48	23.21	25.19	29.59
11	2.603	3.053	3.816	4.575	5.578	7.584	10.34	13.70	17.28	19.68	21.92	24.73	26.76	31.26
12	3.074	3.571	4.404	5.226	6.304	8.438	11.34	14.85	18.55	21.03	23.34	26.22	28.30	32.91
13	3.565	4.107	5.009	5.892	7.042	9.299	12.34	15.98	19.81	22.36	24.74	27.69	29.82	34.53
14	4.075	4.660	5.629	6.571	7.790	10.17	13.34	17.12	21.06	23.68	26.12	29.14	31.32	36.12
15	4.601	5.229	6.262	7.261	8.547	11.04	14.34	18.25	22.31	25.00	27.49	30.58	32.80	37.70
16	5.142	5.812	6.908	7.962	9.312	11.91	15.34	19.37	23.54	26.30	28.85	32.00	34.27	39.25
17	5.697	6.408	7.564	8.672	10.09	12.79	16.34	20.49	24.77	27.59	30.19	33.41	35.72	40.79
18	6.265	7.015	8.231	9.390	10.86	13.68	17.34	21.60	25.99	28.87	31.53	34.81	37.16	42.31
19	6.844	7.633	8.907	10.12	11.65	14.56	18.34	22.72	27.20	30.14	32.85	36.19	38.58	43.82
20	7.434	8.260	9.591	10.85	12.44	15.45	19.34	23.83	28.41	31.41	34.17	37.57	40.00	45.31
21	8.034	8.897	10.28	11.59	13.24	16.34	20.34	24.93	29.62	32.67	35.48	38.93	41.40	46.80
22	8.643	9.542	10.98	12.34	14.04	17.24	21.34	26.04	30.81	33.92	36.78	40.29	42.80	48.27
23	9.260	10.20	11.69	13.09	14.85	18.14	22.34	27.14	32.01	35.17	38.08	41.64	44.18	49.73
24	9.886	10.86	12.40	13.85	15.66	19.04	23.34	28.24	33.20	36.42	39.36	42.98	45.56	51.18
25	10.52	11.52	13.12	14.61	16.47	19.94	24.34	29.34	34.38	37.65	40.65	44.31	46.93	52.62
26	11.16	12.20	13.84	15.38	17.29	20.84	25.34	30.43	35.56	38.89	41.92	45.64	48.29	54.05
27	11.81	12.88	14.57	16.15	18.11	21.75	26.34	31.53	36.74	40.11	43.19	46.96	49.64	55.48
28	12.46	13.56	15.31	16.93	18.94	22.66	27.34	32.62	37.92	41.34	44.46	48.28	50.99	56.89
29	13.12	14.26	16.05	17.71	19.77	23.57	28.34	33.71	39.09	42.56	45.72	49.59	52.34	58.30
30	13.79	14.95	16.79	18.49	20.60	24.48	29.34	34.80	40.26	43.77	46.98	50.89	53.67	59.70
40	20.71	22.16	24.43	26.51	29.05	33.66	39.34	45.62	51.81	55.76	59.34	63.69	66.77	73.40
50	27.99	29.71	32.36	34.76	37.69	42.94	49.33	56.33	63.17	67.50	71.42	76.15	79.49	86.66
60	35.53	37.48	40.48	43.19	46.46	52.29	59.33	66.98	74.40	79.08	83.30	88.38	91.95	99.61
70	43.28	45.44	48.76	51.74	55.33	61.70	69.33	77.58	85.53	90.53	95.02	100.4	104.2	112.3
80	51.17	53.54	57.15	60.39	64.28	71.14	79.33	88.13	96.58	101.9	106.6	112.3	116.3	124.8
90	59.20	61.75	65.65	69.13	73.29	80.62	89.33	98.65	107.6	113.1	118.1	124.1	128.3	137.2
100	67.33	70.06	74.22	77.93	82.36	90.13	99.33	109.1	118.5	124.3	129.6	135.8	140.2	149.4

Table A.2. *Table of critical values of* t

df	Probability								
	.50	.20	.10	.050	.02	.010	.0050	.002	.0010
1	1.000	3.078	6.314	12.71	31.82	63.66	127.3	318.3	636.6
2	0.816	1.886	2.920	4.303	6.965	9.925	14.09	22.33	31.60
3	0.765	1.638	2.353	3.182	4.541	5.841	7.453	10.21	12.92
4	0.741	1.533	2.132	2.776	3.747	4.604	5.598	7.173	8.610
5	0.727	1.476	2.015	2.571	3.365	4.032	4.773	5.893	6.869
6	0.718	1.440	1.943	2.447	3.143	3.707	4.317	5.208	5.959
7	0.711	1.415	1.895	2.365	2.998	3.499	4.029	4.785	5.408
8	0.706	1.397	1.860	2.306	2.896	3.355	3.833	4.501	5.041
9	0.703	1.383	1.833	2.262	2.821	3.250	3.690	4.297	4.781
10	0.700	1.372	1.812	2.228	2.764	3.169	3.581	4.144	4.587
11	0.697	1.363	1.796	2.201	2.718	3.106	3.497	4.025	4.437
12	0.695	1.356	1.782	2.179	2.681	3.055	3.428	3.930	4.318
13	0.694	1.350	1.771	2.160	2.650	3.012	3.372	3.852	4.221
14	0.692	1.345	1.761	2.145	2.624	2.977	3.326	3.787	4.140
15	0.691	1.341	1.753	2.131	2.602	2.947	3.286	3.733	4.073
16	0.690	1.337	1.746	2.120	2.583	2.921	3.252	3.686	4.015
17	0.689	1.333	1.740	2.110	2.567	2.898	3.222	3.646	3.965
18	0.688	1.330	1.734	2.101	2.552	2.878	3.197	3.610	3.922
19	0.688	1.328	1.729	2.093	2.539	2.861	3.174	3.579	3.883
20	0.687	1.325	1.725	2.086	2.528	2.845	3.153	3.552	3.850
21	0.686	1.323	1.721	2.080	2.518	2.831	3.135	3.527	3.819
22	0.686	1.321	1.717	2.074	2.508	2.819	3.119	3.505	3.792
23	0.685	1.319	1.714	2.069	2.500	2.807	3.104	3.485	3.767
24	0.685	1.318	1.711	2.064	2.492	2.797	3.091	3.467	3.745
25	0.684	1.316	1.708	2.060	2.485	2.787	3.078	3.450	3.725
26	0.684	1.315	1.706	2.056	2.479	2.779	3.067	3.435	3.707
27	0.684	1.314	1.703	2.052	2.473	2.771	3.057	3.421	3.690
28	0.683	1.313	1.701	2.048	2.467	2.763	3.047	3.408	3.674
29	0.683	1.311	1.699	2.045	2.462	2.756	3.038	3.396	3.659
30	0.683	1.310	1.697	2.042	2.457	2.750	3.030	3.385	3.646
40	0.681	1.303	1.684	2.021	2.423	2.704	2.971	3.307	3.551
60	0.679	1.296	1.671	2.000	2.390	2.660	2.915	3.232	3.460
120	0.677	1.289	1.658	1.980	2.358	2.617	2.860	3.160	3.373
∞	0.674	1.282	1.645	1.960	2.326	2.576	2.807	3.090	3.291

Source: Biometrika Tables for Statisticians, 3d ed., vol. 1, Table 12.

Table A.3. *Levels of significance of Pearson product-moment correlation coefficients*

df	Probability					
	.20	.10	.05	.02	.01	.002
1	.9511	.9877	.9969	$.9^351$	$.9^388$	$.9^551$
2	.800	.900	.9500	.9800	.9900	.9980
3	.687	.805	.878	.9343	.9587	.9859
4	.608	.729	.811	.882	.9172	.9633
5	.551	.669	.754	.833	.875	.9350
6	.507	.621	.707	.789	.834	.9049
7	.472	.582	.666	.750	.798	.875
8	.443	.549	.632	.715	.765	.847
9	.419	.521	.602	.685	.735	.820
10	.398	.497	.576	.658	.708	.795
11	.380	.476	.553	.634	.684	.772
12	.365	.458	.532	.612	.661	.750
13	.351	.441	.514	.592	.641	.730
14	.338	.426	.497	.574	.623	.711
15	.327	.412	.482	.558	.606	.694
16	.317	.400	.468	.543	.590	.678
17	.308	.389	.456	.529	.575	.662
18	.299	.378	.444	.516	.561	.648
19	.291	.369	.433	.503	.549	.635
20	.284	.360	.423	.492	.537	.622
21	.277	.352	.413	.482	.526	.610
22	.271	.344	.404	.472	.515	.599
23	.265	.337	.396	.462	.505	.588
24	.260	.330	.388	.453	.496	.578
25	.255	.323	.381	.445	.487	.568
26	.250	.317	.374	.437	.479	.559
27	.245	.311	.367	.430	.471	.550
28	.241	.306	.361	.423	.463	.541
29	.237	.301	.355	.416	.456	.533
30	.233	.296	.349	.409	.449	.526
35	.216	.275	.325	.381	.418	.492
40	.202	.257	.304	.358	.393	.463
45	.190	.243	.288	.338	.372	.439
50	.181	.231	.273	.322	.354	.419
60	.165	.211	.250	.295	.325	.385
70	.153	.195	.232	.274	.302	.358
80	.143	.183	.217	.257	.283	.336
90	.135	.173	.205	.242	.267	.318
100	.128	.164	.195	.230	.254	.303
120	.117	.150	.178	.210	.232	.277

Source: From Table VII of R. A. Fisher & F. Yates, *Statistical Tables for Biological, Agricultural and Medical Research,* 6th ed., 1974, published by Longman Group Ltd., London (previously published by Oliver and Boyd Ltd., Edinburgh), and by permission of the authors and publishers.

Table A.4. *Areas under the unit normal curve: for calculating the significance of* z *– the unit normal variate*

z	Probability	z	Probability
0	.500	2.1	.018
.1	.460	2.2	.014
.2	.421	2.3	.011
.3	.382	2.4	.008
.4	.345	2.5	.006
.5	.309	2.6	.005
.6	.274	2.7	.003
.7	.242	2.8	.003
.8	.212	2.9	.002
.9	.184	3.0	.00135
1.0	.159	3.1	.00097
1.1	.136	3.2	.00069
1.2	.115	3.3	.00048
1.3	.097	3.4	.00034
1.4	.081	3.5	.00023
1.5	.067	3.6	.00016
1.6	.055	3.7	.00011
1.7	.045	3.8	.00007
1.8	.036	3.9	.00005
1.9	.029	4.0	.00003
2.0	.023		

Source: Adapted from Table III of R. A. Fisher & F. Yates, *Statistical Tables for Biological, Agricultural and Medical Research,* 6th ed., 1974, published by Longman Group Ltd., London (previously published by Oliver and Boyd Ltd., Edinburgh), and by permission of the authors and publishers.

Table A.5. F ratios for .05 and .01 levels of significance

df for smaller mean square	df for greater mean square									
	1	2	3	4	5	6	8	12	24	∞
1	1.61. / 4052.	200. / 5000.	216. / 5403.	225. / 5625.	230. / 5764.	234. / 5859.	239. / 5981.	244. / 6106.	249. / 6234.	254. / 6366.
2	18.5 / 98.5	19.0 / 99.0	19.2 / 99.2	19.2 / 99.2	19.3 / 99.3	19.3 / 99.3	19.4 / 99.4	19.4 / 99.4	19.5 / 99.5	19.5 / 99.5
3	10.1 / 34.1	9.55 / 30.8	9.28 / 29.5	9.12 / 28.7	9.01 / 28.2	8.94 / 27.9	8.8 / 27.5	8.74 / 27.05	8.64 / 26.6	8.53 / 26.1
4	7.71 / 21.2	6.94 / 18.0	6.59 / 16.7	6.39 / 16.0	6.26 / 15.5	6.16 / 15.2	6.04 / 14.8	5.91 / 14.37	5.77 / 13.9	5.63 / 13.5
5	6.61 / 16.3	5.79 / 13.3	5.41 / 12.1	5.19 / 11.4	5.05 / 11.01	4.95 / 10.7	4.82 / 10.3	4.68 / 9.89	4.53 / 9.47	4.36 / 9.02
6	5.99 / 13.7	5.14 / 10.9	4.76 / 9.78	4.53 / 9.15	4.39 / 8.75	4.28 / 8.47	4.15 / 8.10	4.00 / 7.72	3.84 / 7.31	3.67 / 6.88
7	5.5 / 12.2	4.74 / 9.55	4.35 / 8.45	4.12 / 7.85	3.97 / 7.46	3.87 / 7.19	3.73 / 6.84	3.57 / 6.47	3.41 / 6.07	3.23 / 5.65
8	5.32 / 11.3	4.46 / 8.65	4.07 / 7.59	3.84 / 7.01	3.69 / 6.63	3.58 / 6.37	3.44 / 6.03	3.28 / 5.67	3.12 / 5.28	2.93 / 4.86
9	5.12 / 10.6	4.26 / 8.02	3.86 / 6.66	3.63 / 6.42	3.48 / 6.06	3.37 / 5.80	3.23 / 5.47	3.07 / 5.11	2.90 / 4.73	2.71 / 4.31
10	4.96 / 10.0	4.10 / 7.56	3.71 / 6.55	3.48 / 5.99	3.33 / 5.64	3.22 / 5.39	3.07 / 5.06	2.91 / 4.71	2.74 / 4.33	2.54 / 3.91
11	4.84 / 9.65	3.98 / 7.20	3.59 / 6.22	3.36 / 5.67	3.20 / 5.32	3.09 / 5.07	2.95 / 4.74	2.79 / 4.40	2.61 / 4.02	2.40 / 3.60

Source: Adapted from Biometrika Tables for Statisticians, 3d ed., vol. 1, Table 18.

Table A.6. *Table of critical values of the Spearman rank correlation coefficient (rho)*

	Significance level (one-tailed test)	
N	.05	.01
4	1.000	
5	.900	1.000
6	.829	.943
7	.714	.893
8	.643	.833
9	.600	.783
10	.564	.746
12	.506	.712
14	.456	.645
16	.425	.601
18	.399	.564
20	.377	.534
22	.359	.508
24	.343	.485
26	.329	.465
28	.317	.448
30	.306	.432

Source: Adapted from E. G. Olds, Distributions of sums of squares of rank differences for small numbers of individuals, *Annals of Mathematical Statistics* 9 (1938): 133–148, and from E. G. Olds, The 5% significance levels for sums of squares of rank differences and a correction, ibid. 20 (1949): 117–118, with permission.

Glossary

Analysis of variance (frequently referred to as ANOVA): A method for the simultaneous comparison of many means (*see F* ratio for use on parametrics; Friedman and Kruskal–Wallis tests for non-parametrics)

Arithmetic mean: A measure of central tendency; the sum of a set of values divided by the number of values in the set. Also called the average

Average: *See* Arithmetic mean

Blinding: Keeping the subjects from knowing whether they are in the experimental or the control group

Causal relation research: A concept has reached this stage of research when it fulfills the following criteria:

1. There are (at least) two measured variables
2. The treatment (in the broad sense of the word) is applied to the experimental group of patients/subjects and withheld from the control group. Note that there may be two or more values of the treatment as, for example, different dosages of the same drug. In this case, it is called the treatment variable
3. All possible conditions other than the treatment are held constant so that the control group will be as much like the experimental group as possible, except for the treatment applied by the researcher. If this is done, there is a high probability that any changes in the dependent variable for the experimental group may be attributed to the treatment
4. There must be one or more dependent variables. The dependent variables are those that are observed by the researcher after the treatment is applied. They are measured in both the experimental and control groups to see if the experimental group showed a greater change than the controls

chi-square (χ^2): A nonparametric statistic used to test whether a significant difference exists between an observed number of objects or responses falling in each of two or more categories and an expected number based on the null hypothesis. Also used to test goodness of fit

Cochran Q test: A nonparametric test for use with more than two related samples. Tests whether three or more matched sets of frequencies or proportions differ significantly among themselves. Suitable for data on a nominal scale or for dichotomies

Comparison group: Any group being compared with the experimental group or the group of primary interest

Contingency coefficient (C): A nonparametric measure of the extent of association between two or more sets of attributes

Continuous variable: A variable that may take on any value in a continuous interval of measurement

Control: In statistical parlance, to hold constant or otherwise eliminate

Control group: A group in which all conditions are the same as those for the experimental group except that the treatment is withheld. After the treatment is applied to the experimental group, the values of the dependent variable for experimental subjects are compared with the values of the dependent variable for subjects in the control group to determine whether they are significantly different and can thus be considered to be due to the treatment

Correlation: A measure of degree of association (*see* Kendall rank correlation, Multiple correlation, Product-moment correlation, Spearman rank correlation)

Degrees of freedom *(df)*: The number of comparisons possible given a set of independent means

Dependent variable: The variable in which a change is expected when a treatment is applied to the independent variable

Discrete variable: A variable that can take on only specific values, such as whole numbers, and that has no meaningful values between those numbers (e.g., number of persons)

Double-blinding: Keeping the subjects as well as the persons conducting the experiment from knowing at the time of administration of a treatment whether a given subject is in the experimental or control group

Experiment: A study where the experimenter imposes a systematic change (the treatment) on an independent variable in order to determine its effect on a dependent variable

F ratio: The ratio of one estimate of the variance to another independent estimate of it. Used in analysis of variance. Also called *F* test

F test: *See F* ratio

Factor analysis: A method for determining, by means of a correlational matrix, which of a large number of arbitrarily specified variables may be regarded as the fundamental variables of a set

Fisher exact probability test: A nonparametric test for independent samples. For analyzing discrete data (either nominal or ordinal) when the two independent samples are small in size

Friedman two-way analysis of variance: A nonparametric test for simultaneous comparison of multiple means

Hypothesis: Testable statement of what the experimenter expects the results to be

Incidence: The actual occurrence of an event, such as the numbers and rate of occurrence of a specific disease among patients in a hospital. It is an expression of how much the population utilizes resources

Independent variable: The variable that the experimenter selects or manipulates, and whose effects on the dependent variable he or she determines

Interval scale: A scale where the difference between any two adjacent numbers is the same as the difference between any other two adjacent numbers

Kendall rank correlation coefficient: A nonparametric measure of degree of association between two rank-ordered variables

Kruskall–Wallis one-way analysis of variance: A nonparametric analysis of variance

Latin square design: A method used in analysis of variance for assigning treatments so that one and only one treatment occurs in any one row and in any one column. Hence there must be an equal number of rows, columns, and treatments

Level of significance: The probability with which a given statistical result could have occurred by chance

Likert scale: A commonly used scale for measuring opinions or attitudes that provides anchor points at either end for responses that range from terms like *zero* at the low end to *outstanding* at the high end of the scale, and with rank-ordered points in between

Linear correlation: *See* Correlation

Mann–Whitney U Test: A nonparametric test for independent samples

Matched controls: Control subjects, each of whom is individually matched with a corresponding experimental subject on variables that the experimenter thinks necessary to control (such as age, sex, marital status)

Mean: *See* Arithmetic mean

Mediating variable: A variable appearing between the independent and dependent variables, either naturally or by design

MEDLARS: The Medical Literature Analysis and Retrieval System of the National Library of Medicine. A very useful source of titles for reviewing the medical literature; provides a number of databases in an online computerized network

MEDLINE: The biomedical database of MEDLARS; especially useful for reviewing the current and recent clinical literature

Multiple correlation coefficient (R): The coefficient of correlation between observed scores on some trait and scores predicted for that trait by a multiple regression equation

Multiple regression: *See* Regression equation

Needs assessment: In psychiatric use, a determination by means of quantitative research of the treatment requirements of a patient, the programmatic requirements of a hospital or treatment unit, or the inpatient, outpatient, partial hospitalization, etc. requirements of a community

Nominal scale: A scale where numbers or other symbols are used simply to classify objects. Measurement at its weakest level

Nonparametric statistics: A wide variety of statistics not based upon an underlying assumption of a normally distributed population variable for use with variables measured on nominal, ordinal, or interval scales. Also called distribution-free statistics. (*See,* for example, in any statistical text containing nonparametric statistics, Binomial test, Cochran Q test for related samples, Fisher exact probability test, Kendall rank correlation coefficient, Kolmogorov–Smirnov one-sample test, Kruskal–Wallis one-way analysis of variance, Mann–Whitney U Test for independent samples, Sign test, Spearman rank correlation coefficient, Walsh test for related samples, Wilcoxon matched-pairs signed-ranks test for related samples)

Observed causal research: A concept has reached this stage of research when it fulfills the following criteria:

1. There are (at least) two measured variables
2. There are two or more values of a treatment variable, which may or may not be under the control of the experimenter
3. There are one or more dependent variables. There must be two (or

more) measures of each dependent variable, corresponding to two (or more) values of the treatment variable

Observed relation research: A concept has reached this stage of research when it fulfills the following criteria:

1. There are at least two measurements on each of two (or more) measured variables
2. These variables are observed for concomitant variation
3. Other factors (known or unknown) may or may not be held constant

Operational definition: A definition of a concept expressed in terms of an operation or procedure. For example, anxiety can be defined operationally with a description in the APA's *Diagnostic and Statistical Manual of Mental Disorders* or with a score on a test for measuring anxiety

Ordinal scale: A group of items such that each member of the group stands in some relationship to the others in terms of greater than, more difficult than, sicker than, and so on, but where it is impossible to quantify the amount by which one item exceeds another in this quality

Parameter: In statistics, the value of a variable (such as the mean or variance) for the entire population (as compared with a sample value, which is called a statistic)

Parametric statistics: Statistics based on the assumption of an underlying population with a defined distribution (usually the normal distribution)

Phi coefficient (ϕ): A nonparametric index of strength of association

Placebo effect: The psychological effect obtained when subjects are administered an innocuous substance that they believe to be a therapeutic treatment

Population: In statistics, the group of all members having a defined characteristic or set of characteristics

Power of a statistical test: The probability that a statistical test will give a significant difference when a difference exists in the sample

Prevalence: The degree to which a population is affected with a particular disease at a given time; the percentage or rate of occurrence of the disease in the population as a whole. Prevalence indicates the population's need for services

Probability of occurrence by chance (p): The probability that if the same experiment (or test or comparison) were repeated a given number of times, the obtained result would have occurred purely by chance

Probit analysis: A procedure used in demand forecasting that follows the principle of maximum likelihood rather than that of least squares. Its mathematical derivation is fairly complex

Product-moment correlation (*r*): A parametric statistic that reflects the degree of association between two sets of measurements, using a zero value to indicate no relationship, and a plus or minus 1 to indicate perfect correlation, the minus indicating the inverse relationship between the two number scales used. Also called the Pearson *r*

Random assignment: Assignment of subjects to two or more groups in a way such that each subject has the same chance of being assigned to any one group (assignment by deciding that every other subject should go into the control group is not random assignment; nor is selection of even-numbered individuals for experimentals and odd-numbered ones for controls)

Random selection: Selection of subjects in such a way that every subject in the population has the same probability of being selected to be a member of the sample. Ideally, this is done by assigning a number to each member of the population and then selecting subjects by referring to consecutive numbers in a table of random numbers such as usually appears in the back of a statistical text. When there is a large pool of subjects available for research, this is the method used in order to avoid biasing the results by any other selection method

Randomized block design: A method used in analysis of variance in which the order of treatment is randomized to remove the effect of individual differences and order of presentation of the treatments

Rank order correlation: Correlation between two sets of numbers each of which was derived from scores on a rank-ordered scale (*see* Kendall rank correlation coefficient, Spearman rank correlation coefficient)

Ratio scale: A scale having all the properties of an interval scale and in addition having a true zero point. A scale isomorphic to the structure of arithmetic. Highest level of measurement

Regression equation: An equation of the type $Y = a + bx$, where Y is a criterion, a is a constant, b is the regression coefficient, and x is a predictor variable. Used to predict changes in Y from changes in x. When there is more than one x variable from which Y is to be predicted, called a multiple regression equation

Reliability: The degree to which a clinical test consistently measures the same objects or events as long as it is administered, from beginning to end, and yields the same results consistently when repeated under the same conditions

Research to develop measuring instruments (the second stage of research): A concept has reached this stage of research if it fulfills the following criteria:

1. It can be defined in words
2. There exists a specifiable technique for measuring it, an operational definition
3. There is agreement on the outcomes of measurement. It has won acceptance because it has been shown to be reliable

Research to formulate an initial working hypothesis (the first stage of research): An initial working hypothesis is one in which not all the terms have yet been defined operationally and the relationship expressed has not been demonstrated. The statement has been arrived at through personal impression, experience, or discussion

Sample: In statistics, a randomly selected group of subjects from a given population

Selectivity: Selectivity relates to a clinical test's ability to confirm the absence of a disease in patients who do not have it, and to avoid a false positive

Sensitivity: Sensitivity refers to a clinical test's ability to diagnose the presence of the disease in patients who actually have it, and to avoid false negatives

Sign test: A nonparametric test for related samples. Uses plus and minus signs rather than quantitative measures as its data. Useful for research in which quantitative measurement is impossible or infeasible, but in which it is possible to rank the two members of each pair with respect to each other

Significance of a difference: The probability (p) that an observed difference could have occurred by chance

Spearman rank correlation coefficient: *See* Rank-order correlation coefficient

Specificity of a test: The extent to which one of a battery of tests measures a factor not measured by any of the other tests; the opposite of homogeneity. A test should be internally homogeneous, i.e., each item should be a slightly different measurement of the same variable. For a battery of tests (e.g., to measure liver function or emotional depression), the greatest economy is achieved if each test has high specificity and measures a different factor or variable

Standard deviation *(SD)*: A measure of the dispersion of scores about the mean of a distribution; the square root of the variance

Standard score, standardized score: A linear transformation of a raw score into a set of scores whose mean is 0 and whose standard deviation is 1. Usually called *z* scores. This procedure is used to make diverse scores from different tests comparable

Standardized test: A test with known validity and reliability

Statistic: A sample value (as contrasted to a parameter, which is a population value)

Statistical test: A test of the probability of a significant difference between two statistics derived from random samples

Student's *t* test: A parametric test of the significance of a difference between two sample means ("Student" is the pseudonym of the test's inventor)

Subject: In research, a member of a group being observed, tested, or measured

t test: *See* Student's *t* test

Theory development: A theory provides a description or operational definition of how to classify, predict, or control events. A theoretical article integrates research findings; it need not present original data. It is based on measurement, observed relation, and causal relation researches. A theory's principal characteristic is that it summarizes the results of several researches and attempts to make generalizations based on their findings

Treatment: In statistics, any change applied by the experimenter to the independent variable in order to assess expected effects on the dependent variable

Treatment variable: A treatment having two or more values

Validity: The degree to which a test measures what it purports to measure

Variable: A characteristic that may take on several values

Variance: In statistics, the average of the sums of squares of the deviations from the mean of a distribution; the square of the standard deviation

Walsh test: A nonparametric test for related samples

Wilcoxon matched-pairs signed-ranks test: A nonparametric test for use with related samples. Makes use of direction (plus or minus) and relative magnitude of differences within pairs

References

Albee, G. W. 1982. Preventing psychopathology and promoting human potential. *American Psychologist* 37: 1043–1050.

Alderman, A. A., Gordon, R. E., Gordon, K. K., Ahsanuddin, K. M. & Slaymaker, C. J. 1984. Functional Level Equation in comprehensive treatment planning. *Bulletin of Southern Psychiatry* 3,2: 10–21.

American Psychiatric Association. 1980. *Diagnostic and Statistical Manual of Mental Disorders,* 3d ed. *(DSM-III).* Washington, DC: Author. 3d ed. revised, 1987.

Aumack, L. 1962. Social Adjustment Behavior Rating Scale (SABRS). *Journal of Clinical Psychology* 13: 436–441.

Beck, A. T. 1972. Measuring depression: the depression inventory. In T. Williams, M. M. Katz & J. A. Shield (eds.), *Recent Advances in the Psychobiology of the Depressive Illnesses.* Washington, DC: Government Printing Office.

Boston Women's Health Book Collective. 1973. *Our Bodies, Ourselves: A Book by and for Women.* New York: Simon & Schuster.

Brooks, G. W. & Mueller, E. 1966. Serum urate concentrations among professors. *Journal of the American Medical Association* 195: 416.

Burdock, E. I. & Hardesty, A. S. 1969. *The Structured Clinical Interview (SCI).* New York: Springer.

Caton, C. L. & Gralnick, A. 1987. A review of the issues surrounding length of psychiatric hospitalization. *Hospital and Community Psychiatry* 38: 858–863.

Clark, E. M. & Gordon, R. E. 1970. Polyphasic health testing – its service to Florida physicians. *Journal of the Florida Medical Association* 57: 24–27, 197.

Cogan, R. 1980. Postpartum depression. *International Childbirth Education Association Review* 4: 1–5.

Cohen, M., Gordon, R. E., Adams, J., Marlowe, H., Bedell, J. & Weathers, L. 1979. Single bedtime dose self-medication system. *Hospital and Community Psychiatry* 30: 30–33.

Edmunson, E. D., Bedell, J., Archer, R. & Gordon, R. E. 1982. Integrating skill building and peer support in mental health treatment. In A. Jeger & R. Slotnick (eds.), *Community Mental Health and Behavioral Ecology,* pp. 127–139. New York: Plenum.

Edmunson, E. D., Bedell, J. & Gordon, R. E. 1984. Bridging the gap between professional aftercare and peer support. In A. Gartner & F. Riessman (eds.), *The Self-Help Revolution,* pp. 195–203. New York: Human Science Press.

Feldman, D. & Gagnon, J. 1985. StatView. Calabasas, CA: BrainPower, Inc.

Finkelstein, M. 1985. *Statistics at Your Fingertips.* Belmont, CA: Wadsworth.

Gartner, A. J. & Riessman, F. 1982. Self-help and mental health. *Hospital and Community Psychiatry* 33: 631–635.

Gordon, K. K. & Gordon, R. E. 1964. Folk healers and modern medicine. *Journal of the American Medical Association* 189: 238–239.

Gordon, R. E. 1959. Sociodynamics and psychotherapy. *A.M.A. Archives of Neurology and Psychiatry* 81: 486–503.

Gordon, R. E. 1961. *Prevention of Postpartum Emotional Difficulties.* Ann Arbor, MI: University Microfilms.

Gordon, R. E. 1966. Is short-term psychotherapy enough? *Journal of the Medical Society of New Jersey* 63: 41–44.

Gordon, R. E. 1971. Psychiatric screening through multiphasic health testing. *American Journal of Psychiatry* 128: 51–55.

Gordon, R. E., Bielen, L. & Watts, A. M. 1973. Psychiatric screening utilizing automated multiphasic testing in the VA admission procedure. *American Journal of Psychiatry* 130: 46–48.

Gordon, R. E., Edmunson, E. D., Archer, R. & Weinberg, R. 1981. *The use of networks and social support in therapy.* Course presented at the 133d Annual Meeting, American Psychiatric Association, San Francisco.

Gordon, R. E. & Gordon, K. K. 1959. Psychosomatic problems of a rapidly growing suburb. *Journal of the American Medical Association* 169: 16.

Gordon, R. E. & Gordon, K. K. 1960. Social factors in the prevention of postpartum emotional problems. *Obstetrics and Gynecology* 15: 443–448.

Gordon, R. E. & Gordon, K. K. 1963. *The Blight on the Ivy.* Englewood Cliffs, NJ: Prentice-Hall.

Gordon, R. E. & Gordon, K. K. 1981. *Systems of Treatment for the Mentally Ill: Filling the Gaps.* New York: Grune and Stratton.

Gordon, R. E. & Gordon, K. K. 1982. The FL-Equation and professional roles in psychiatry. *Bulletin of Southern Psychiatry* 1,1: 13–14.

Gordon, R. E. & Gordon, K. K. 1983. Predicting length of hospitalization with diagnostically related groups of psychiatric patients. *Bulletin of Southern Psychiatry* 2,4: 13–20.

Gordon, R. E. & Gordon, K. K. 1985. A program of modular psychoeducational skills training for chronic mental patients. In L. L'Abate & M. A. Milan (eds.), *Handbook of Social Skills Training and Research,* pp. 388–417. New York: Wiley.

Gordon, R. E. & Gordon, K. K. 1987. Relating Axes IV and V of DSM-III to clinical severity of psychiatric disorders. *Canadian Journal of Psychiatry* 32: 423–424.

Gordon, R. E., Gordon, K. K., Gordon-Hardy, L. L., Hursch, C. J. & Reed, K. G. 1986. Predicting perinatal emotional adjustment with psychosocial and hormonal measures in early pregnancy. *American Journal of Obstetrics and Gynecology* 155: 80–82.

Gordon, R. E., Gordon, K. K. & Gunther, M. 1961. *The Split-Level Trap.* New York: Geis.

Gordon, R. E. Gordon, K. K., Plutzky, M. & Guerra, M. In press. Using the Axis V scale to measure therapeutic outcome of psychiatric treatment. *Canadian Journal of Psychiatry.*

Gordon, R. E., Holzer, C., Bielen, L., Watts, A. M. & Gordon, K. L. 1973. AMHTS and VA admission procedure. In Dean F. Davies (ed.), *Health Evaluation.* New York: Intercontinental Medical.

Gordon, R. E., Jardiolin, P. & Gordon, K. K. 1985. Predicting length of hospital stay of psychiatric patients. *American Journal of Psychiatry* 142: 235–237.

Gordon, R. E., Kapostins, E. E. & Gordon, K. K. 1960. Electroencephalographic and social psychological indicators of nursing student performance. *Nursing Research* 9: 1.

Gordon, R. E., Kapostins, E. E. & Gordon, K. K. 1965. Factors in postpartum emotional adjustment. *Obstetrics and Gynecology* 25: 156–166.

Gordon, R. E., Lindeman, R. H. & Gordon, K. K. 1967. Some psychological and chemical correlates of college achievement. *College Health* 15: 326–331.

Gordon, R. E., Lyons, H. R., Muniz, C. & Most, B. 1973. The migratory disabled veteran. *Journal of the Florida Medical Association* 60: 27–30.

Gordon, R. E., McWhorter, J. E., Singer, M. G. & Gordon, K. K. 1960. Coronary artery disease in a rapidly growing suburb. *Journal of the Medical Society of New Jersey* 57: 677–683.

Gordon, R. E., Patterson, R. L., Eberly, D. A. & Penner, L. A. 1980. Modular treatment of psychiatric patients. In J. H. Masserman (ed.), *Current Psychiatric Therapies,* New York: Grune and Stratton.

Gordon, R. E., Singer, M. G. & Gordon, K. K. 1961. Social psychological stress. *Archives of General Psychiatry* 4: 459.

Gordon, R. E., Singer, M. G. & Gordon, K. K. 1962. The stress of obtaining a higher education. *Journal of the Medical Society of New Jersey* 59: 608–614.

Gordon, R. E., Vijay, J., Sloate, S. G., Burket, R. & Gordon, K. K. 1985. Aggravating stress and functional level as predictors of length of psychiatric hospitalization. *Hospital and Community Psychiatry* 36: 773–774.

Gordon, R. E., Warheit, G. J., Hursch, C. J., Schwab, J. J., Watts, A. M. & Gordon, K. L. 1975. Sorting out the worried well from the really sick. *Medical Times* 102: 97.

Gordon, R. E. & Webb, S. 1975. The orbiting psychiatric patient. *Journal of the Florida Medical Association* 62: 21–25.

Greene, R. L. 1980. *The MMPI: An Interpretive Manual.* Orlando, FL: Grune & Stratton.

Hamilton, M. 1959. The assessment of anxiety states by rating. *British Journal of Medical Psychology* 32: 50.

Hamilton, M. 1960. A rating scale for depression. *Journal of Neurology, Neurosurgery and Psychiatry* 23: 56–62.

Hammond, K. R., Hursch, C. J. & Todd, F. J. 1964. Analyzing the components of clinical inference. *Psychological Review* 71: 438–456.

Heim, N. & Hursch, C. J. 1979. Castration for sex offenders – treatment or punishment. *Archives of Sexual Behavior* 8,3: 281–304.

Hogarty, G. E. & Ulrich, R. 1972. The discharge readiness inventory. *Archives of General Psychiatry* 26: 419–426.

Hokanson, J. A., Bryant, S. G., Gardner, R., Luttman, D. J., Guernsey, B. G. & Bienkowski, A. C. 1986. Spectrum and frequency of use of statistical techniques in psychiatric journals. *American Journal of Psychiatry* 143: 1118–1125.

Hollingshead, A. B. & Redlich, F. C. 1958. *Social Class and Mental Illness: Community Study.* New York: Wiley.

Holmes, T. H. & Rahe, R. H. 1967. The social adjustment rating scale. *Journal of Psychosomatic Research* 11: 213–218.

Honigfeld, G., Gillis, R. & Klett, C. J. 1966. NOSIE-30: A treatment-sensitive ward behavior scale. *Psychological Reports* 19: 180.

Hopkins, J., Marcus, M. & Campbell, S. 1984. Postpartum depression. *Psychological Bulletin* 95: 498–515.

Horst, P. 1966. *Psychological Measurement and Prediction.* Belmont, CA: Wadsworth.

Hursch, C. J. 1970. The scientific study of sleep and dreams. In E. Hartmann (ed.), *International Psychiatry Clinics* 7: 387–402. Boston: Little, Brown.

Hursch, C. J. 1977. *The Trouble with Rape.* Chicago: Nelson Hall.

Hursch, C. J., Karacan, I. & Williams, R. L. 1972. Some characteristics of nocturnal penile tumescence in early middle-aged males. *Comprehensive Psychiatry* 13: 539–548.

Karacan, I., Williams, R. L., Hursch, C. J., McCaulley, M. & Heine, W. 1969. Some implications of the sleep patterns of pregnancy for postpartum emotional disturbances. *British Journal of Psychiatry* 115: 929–935.

Karacan, I., Williams, R. L., Salis, P. J. & Hursch, C. J. 1971. New approaches to the evaluation and treatment of insomnia. *Psychosomatics* 12: 81–88.

Karoly, P. (ed.). 1985. *Measurement Strategies in Health Psychology.* New York: Wiley.

Kasl, S. V., Brooks, G. W. & Cobb, S. 1966. Serum urate concentrations in male high school students, a predictor of college attendance. *Journal of the American Medical Association* 198: 713–716.

Katz, M. M. & Lyerly, S. B. 1963. Methods for measuring adjustment in the community. 1. Rationale, description, discriminative validity and scale development. *Psychological Review* 13: 503.

Lambert, M. J., Christensen, E. R. & DeJulio, S. S. (eds.). 1983. *The Assessment of Psychotherapy Outcome.* New York: Wiley.

Larsen, V., Evans, T., Brodsack, J., Dungey, L., Elliott, J., Harmon, J., Kaess, D., Kaess, S., Karman, I., Main, D., Martin, L., Ramer, J. & Pearson, J. W. 1966. *Attitudes and Stresses Affecting Perinatal Adjustment.* Final Report, NIMH Grant MH–01381–01–02. Fort Steilacoom, WA: Mental Health Research Institute.

Leighton, D. C. 1963. *The Character of Danger.* New York: Basic.

Lindeman, R. H., Gordon, R. E. & Gordon, K. K. 1969. Further relationships between blood chemicals and college student performance and attitudes. *College Health* 18: 156–161.

Lorr, M. 1953. *Multidimensional scale for rating psychiatric patients.* Veterans Administration Technical Bulletin TB 10–507.

Martin, D. W. 1985. *Doing Psychology Experiments.* 2d ed. Monterey, CA: Brooks/Cole.

McBurney, D. H. 1983. *Experimental Psychology.* Belmont, CA: Wadsworth.

Meldman, M. J., McFarland, G. & Johnson, E. 1976. *The Problem-Oriented Psychiatric Index and Treatment Plans.* St. Louis: Mosby.

Ogburn, B., Bellino, R., Williams, R. L. & Gordon, R. E. 1969. Problems of the military retiree. *Journal of the Florida Medical Association* 56: 245–248.

Overall, J. E. & Gorham, D. R. 1962. The Brief Psychiatric Rating Scale. *Psychological Reports* 10: 799.

Patterson, R. L. 1982. *Overcoming the Deficits of Aging.* New York: Plenum.

Pattison, E. M. 1977. Clinical social systems interventions. *Psychiatry Digest* 38: 25–33.

Price, R. H. & Moos, R. H. 1975. Toward a taxonomy of inpatients' treatment environments. *Journal of Abnormal Psychology* 84: 181–188.

Robins, L. N., Helzer, J. E., Croughan, J. & Ratcliff, K. 1981. National Institute of Mental Health Diagnostic Interview Schedule. *Archives of General Psychiatry* 38: 381–389.

Runyon, R. P. 1985. *Fundamentals of Statistics in the Biological, Medical, and Health Sciences.* Boston: Duxbury.

Siegel, S. 1957. *Nonparametric Statistics for the Behavioral Sciences.* New York: McGraw-Hill.

Slater, A., Gordon, K. K. & Gordon, R. E. 1978. Role differences of mental health workers: observations of four sites. In K. B. Nash, N. Lifton & S. E. Smith, (eds.), *The Paraprofessional: Selected Readings.* New Haven, CT: Advocate Press.

Slater, A., Gordon, K., Patterson, R. & Bowman, L. 1978. *Deinstitutionalizing the Elderly in Florida's State Mental Hospitals: Addressing the Problems.* Monograph series no. 2. Tampa, FL: Human Resources Institute, University of South Florida.

Spielberger, C. D. 1968. *The State–Trait Anxiety Inventory.* Palo Alto, CA: Consulting Psychologists Press.

Tolsdorf, C. 1976. Social networks, support and coping. *Family Process* 15: 407–417.

Williams, J. H. 1974. *Psychology of Women: Behavior in a Biosocial Context.* New York: Norton.

Williams, R. L., Hursch, C. J. & Karacan, I. 1972. Between subject variability and night-to-night variability in insomniacs and normal controls. *Sleep Research* 1: 154.

Williams, R. L., Karacan, I. & Hursch, C. J. 1974. *The EEG of Normal Sleep.* New York: Wiley.

Wittenborn, J. R. 1950. A new procedure for evaluating mental hospital patients. *Journal of Consulting and Clinical Psychology* 14: 500.

Wyatt, R. J. 1986. Scienceless to homeless. *Science* 234: 1309.

Index

ABA, ABAB, *see under* design, research
abstract, *see under* format
aggravating stress, *see* stress, aggravating
analysis of variance (ANOVA), 151–3
article, rejected, 9, 30
assessment (*see also* instrument, measuring), 189–91, 193–8, 226, 229, 230; of needs, 102–8, 124–7, 141, 144, 170
assignment, random, *see* selection
Axes IV and V, see under *DSM-III)*

baseline, 39–40, 134 *(fig.)*
bias, 40, 57, 75, 100, 145, 155
bibliography, *see under* format
biomedical impairments, 175–7, 195, 199–200
blinding, 40, 155–6, 168
block design, 150

causal relation research, *see under* stage of research
cause, causality, 11, 93–4, 115, 138–9, 141–2
cell, 43, 161–2
central tendency, 21–4
chi-square (χ^2), 67–72, 79–80, 83–9, 138, 157–68, 236 *(table)*
classification, *see* theory
consent, informed, 44, 216
consultant (*see also* expert), 102, 108, 114, 151, 153–4, 232
contingency coefficient, *see under* correlation
control, *see* theory
controls (*see also* group(s): control), patients as their own, 123–4, 150; waiting list, 123
coping skills, *see* skills: coping
correlation, 93; contingency coefficient, 67, 79–80, 89, 161, 162; multiple (R), 109–10; Pearson's product-moment (r),

108, 116, 119, 238 *(table)*; phi coefficient (ϕ), 67, 72, 80, 83–4; point biserial, 108; Spearman's rank (rho), 67, 102, 116–18, 241 *(table)*; tetrachoric, 108
crossover, 150, 155
cross-validation, 54, 79
curve, normal, 25–7

data, 20–5, 226–7; collection, 59–61, 97–106, 133–8; pooled, 211
definition, operational, 13, 82, 152, 167
degrees of freedom, 71, 83
Delphi method, 98
design, research, 39–41, 123–4, 129–31, 147–8, 150–7; ABA, ABAB, 39–40, 43; Greco-Latin, 151; Latin square, 151; randomized block, 150
deviation, standard, 66, 89–91, 207
directive power, *see* power, directive
discriminant analysis, 108–9
discussion, *see under* format
disease, 80–1, 97–8
double-blinding, *see* blinding
DSM-III (Diagnostic and Statistical Manual of Mental Disorders), 4, 5–6, 13, 64, 145, 217; Axes IV and V, 15, 61–2, 94–5, 176, 180–1, 187–8; *DSM-III-R*, 211–12, 226

environmental supports, *see* supports, environmental
epidemiology, 97–102
ethics, 214–22
evaluation, program, 124–8, 141–9, 159–61, 210–11, 216, 230–1
experimentals, *see* group(s): experimental
expert (*see also* consultant), 47, 75, 98, 103, 163

F test, 153, 240 *(table)*
factor analysis, 109

255

DATE DUE